Hooked?

NET: the new approach to drug cure

Meg Patterson, MBE, MBChB, FRCSE

ISBN: 1-59048-244-1

The Long Riders' Guild Press

To Lorne, Sean and Myrrh
for sharing all the struggles with patience,
understanding, and, now, their lives.

To be hooked: ... More recently it also means addicted to the use of a drug.

Bartlett's Familiar Quotations

addict: addictus: past participle:
addicere: to favour, to adjudge.
(i) to award by judicial decree; (ii) to surrender, to attach oneself as a follower to a person, or adherent to a cause; (iii) to surrender as a constant practice, e.g., 'we sincerely addict ourselves to Almighty God.'
Thomas Fuller.

Webster's Dictionary

Contents

List of Figures (graphs)

Preface

This book is about healing people of their addiction to various kinds of drugs. The title comes from two British Broadcasting Corporation television documentaries, 'Off The Hook' (1975) and 'Still Off The Hook' (1977). The two films followed an officially registered drug addict from the first day of his NeuroElectric Therapy (NET) to the tenth day, then presented a profile of the same individual two years later. A third BBC-TV documentary about NET, 'The Black Box', produced by a scientific rather than a human interest film unit, was broadcast in February 1981.

The book is divided into three parts. Part I addresses the problems associated with detoxification of substance abuse and gives a lay description of NeuroElectric Therapy (NET). Part II explores the scientific rationale behind NET; it also includes an analysis and follow-up of NET-treated patients over seven years in Britain. Part III deals with the psycho-spiritual problems contributing to addiction and the psycho-spiritual solutions. [Readers may choose the part that is most relevant to their particular field of interest.]

There is a curious dichotomy associated with the word 'cure' when applied to addictions – even by doctors. When the question of cure is raised in conditions other than addictions – the common cold or hepatitis for example – it is usually taken by all concerned to mean the temporary resolution of the condition. That is, the cold is treated with medication and disappears for a month or a year, when it may appear again; and the hepatitis is treated and may reappear if the patient again uses dirty needles. Such qualifications are rarely considered by doctors, patients, and the general public when the subject is the cure of addiction, where it is taken by all to mean 'a total cure of all signs of the condition, with no possible recurrence no matter what the patient chooses to do'.

However, in this book the word 'cure' may be defined in two ways. Firstly, the process of detoxification from all substance abuse which can be achieved quickly and with a minimal amount of discomfort, according to all acceptable definitions of 'cure' – medical, scientific and statistical. However, if the addiction condition is expanded to include contributory psycho-spiritual causes, then a number of other factors must be included as criteria in defining 'cure'. Some of these are dealt with in Part III, 'Psychotherapeutic problems and psycho-spiritual solutions'.

The definition of cure for which I would prefer to be judged is the healing in body, mind and spirit, of those who were previously unable to function responsibly because of substance abuse. This would involve a comprehension and a demonstrated capacity to put into effect a new philosophy of life which is adequate to their chosen environment so that they are no longer in bondage to a chemical or behavioural addiction, but can live with freedom, joy and love in family and community.

The treatment of chemical-substance abuse portrayed in the three BBC-TV documentaries, and described in this book, is a demonstrably successful form of therapy discovered in Hong Kong and developed in England. Yet the three documentaries also revealed a conspicuous disinterest in NeuroElectric Therapy by the British government. To develop NET to its present state I have had to turn to private citizens and to private industry for support.

I am grateful to the many scientists who have encouraged and advised me. I also wish to render thanks to the Rank Foundation for funding the clinical trial at the Pharmakon Clinic in Sussex, and to Norman Stone whose BBC films made the Foundation's chairman, Major Cowen, aware of this treatment; to the Clinic staff for their dedication and enthusiasm; to Olivia Timbs for her editorial assistance; to *Omni* magazine for permission to reproduce an article on NET, and especially to the author, Kathleen McAuliffe, for her long and painstaking research before she decided that NET was a valid treatment which should be publicized; to all my patients – for each one of you has taught me something about NET and life; to many friends who have given us practical support and encouragement, particularly the rock music group The Who, and to their leader Pete Townshend for his courage in speaking publicly of his own problems and of his treatment by NET with openness and insight; and, most of all, to my husband George, for his unfailing support and inspiration and his contributions to several chapters.

Somehow, it was appropriate that it was in Hong Kong, and

China, that this treatment was discovered, for it was from Hong Kong in the nineteenth century that the British authorities and traders carried the opium that was to corrupt and destroy the lives of many millions in China. In the twentieth century the possible cure for that addiction has been brought from China to Hong Kong and back to Britain.

So the 'thousand-league journey' which began with the 'one step' in Hong Kong in 1972 is nearing completion, and I would like to thank all those who made the journey possible and memorable. They are still helping and, like myself, experiencing the rewards promised to those who pursue a distant vision with faith and commitment. But many others will be needed to complete the task: the transformation of an uncaring, materialist society into one with compassionate spiritual vision and values.

Meg Patterson
LONDON 1985

I ADDICTION AND POSSIBLE CURE

Introduction
Description of an illicit and a licit addiction

Heroin

Pamela, 23 years old, had been injecting heroin since she was aged 17. She gave this interview three weeks after completing a 10-day treatment by NET.

> I started with pot when I was 15 and then took heroin when I was 17. I am a really indulgent person so I went rapidly downhill. I have never done anything in moderation.
>
> I forged my mother's cheques. I stole from my family and sometimes my boyfriend and I sold heroin.
>
> My father has not lived at home for several years and even when he was there he might as well not have been there; I sometimes wonder if he had been it would have made a difference. He was only brought in for financial reasons.
>
> He likes children in principle – they are proof of his manliness. But I felt terribly rejected by him. He used to say: 'Why are these children here, why are their friends over, why are they having birthday parties?'
>
> You can see that he's lonely now. He's married a woman he wished he hadn't. He has lost contact with his children. My father drinks every night say, six or seven gins. I am not sure whether he is an alcoholic but I'd like to see what would happen if you took his drink away.
>
> My mother's great. She is marvellous but she does make me feel inadequate. I have been too spoilt and indulged by my mother and father: my father through his guilt.
>
> My brother is a paraplegic. He broke his neck in a horse riding accident, three years ago. How can a God let that happen? He's beautiful. He didn't smoke, he didn't drink. He was good at sport; he had a beautiful girlfriend, but he is an embittered person.
>
> I have tried everything to get off heroin: long-term programmes, detox programmes (where they'd dry you out), psychiatrists, hypnotherapy, primal therapy. I was always being sent away. I'd detox

and then within weeks or months I'd start again. It was a continual round of getting money and scoring, getting money and scoring.

Then nearly three years ago I became pregnant: all by mistake. I had never been pregnant before and I couldn't bring myself to have an abortion. Financially there would be no problem. I knew I would have to support the child but I was prepared to do that.

And I thought if I have this baby it will cure me. But it was just the wrong idea. It didn't. I thought if I had something to love me back it would be fine. But it doesn't work like that. I was simply taken up with the whole business of this thing growing inside me. I was on methadone when I was seven months pregnant. The baby had to be detoxified after birth.

I thought having the baby would make me better - his life would save mine.

I came off methadone when the baby was six weeks old. At the time my boyfriend was in this detox programme and said the family should be together. And I went but I couldn't feed the baby, people were shouting all the time. You weren't meant to leave but after a week I sneaked out with the baby. I went back on methadone but that was difficult: it is just meant for pregnant women and really desperate cases. So soon I was using heroin again.

For years and years I had only been scoring £35 at a time, that was it. But recently I was scoring £100 a day.

You know I died in a railway lavatory three months ago. I was found with my feet sticking out. The girl I had been scoring with had stolen my money and gone. I died twice for three minutes, each time, they said. When I came round I first thought of the baby. What have I done? I can't die now. I have another person's life I'm responsible for. How selfish. It was the first time I realized he wasn't just this cute little thing; that I was more involved than that. I had over-dosed before many times - always through carelessness. It was more scary for the family than me. I haven't the guts to slash my wrists. Death is the coward's way out.

It now matters to me that *I* should look after the baby. I want to be my child's mother. I've still got him.

NET was my last chance. Wanting heroin is like having an emotion without thinking. You can't avoid it by running away. It helps the urge for oblivion. I have always been such a great disappointment to myself.

NET was not very different from the times I have cold-turkeyed. The only difference was that the machine took away all the anxiety. You can cope with aching arms and legs and streaming nose but the worst part is the anxiety. Just like before a race or an exam when you get butterflies. Your stomach is churning and churning.

Normally it drives you berserk so it pushes you until you go out and score again.

This time my stomach was completely settled, I didn't feel jumpy or nervous. I felt a little bit sick but more or less normal. I was more interested in what was going on around. It was much less bad than I expected and brilliant compared with other times. It normally lasts seven to ten days.

I know the cure is not everything, it is what happens afterwards. So how can I fill those 24 hours that I used to spend scoring? Up until now I have been comfortable in failure. Maybe it is because I feel safer being a failure; an idiot on the dole. I have got to get over that. I cannot go back to what I was doing. I portray myself as being strong but then why am I so pathetic and a drug addict?

I intend to look after the baby. I would like to be a researcher, do a course. Start taking exercise. But then can I?

The only people who have been successfully straight believe in God, but I am an atheist through and through. I am totally faithless.

I definitely have to believe in something. God is a long way off for me. I try to believe in the baby. Something other than believing in nothing.

If I were Meg I'd be extremely proud to have brought up three children like that. It is wonderful to see a happy affectionate family. A real family. We are just a lot of individuals living in the same house. There is no real closeness.

It freaks me out the idea of bringing the baby up to be a whole person. Someone who is strong and who doesn't need drugs, that he won't grow up weak. That worries me a lot.

The most awful thing out of the whole business is not to be trusted. My family trust me with their lives but not their wallets. I have got to rebuild that trust and it is going to be so difficult.

Ativan

Susan, in her late 30s, recalled her 10-year experience with tranquillizers, three months after treatment by NET.

It was 1973 that I found myself in a doctor's surgery complaining of panic attacks and feelings of depression and confusion. I had just moved from the north of England to London with my husband and two children to start a film course. I was overworking, getting something like four hours sleep a night. In short, I was driving myself too hard.

Looking back, I know that I should have been ordered to rest for a few weeks. Instead, I was given a drug that was to affect my life in the most devastating way. I will never forget that first prescription. After a fairly lengthy discussion, the doctor decided to give me Ativan which he insisted was 'harmless and non-addictive'. Knowing nothing of these matters, I trusted in his professional wisdom. Why not? He knew best.

After a few weeks of dutifully swallowing 6 mg of Ativan a day (six tablets), I realized that there was no way I could function without them. The panic attacks and dizzy spells would return the moment I hadn't got my quota of blue pills in me. A few months after that first prescription I had to ask my doctor for six weeks' supply as I was going on holiday to Morocco with my children. I must have caught him at a bad moment. He shouted down the phone at me something about 'bloody drug addicts'. I slammed the phone down and from then on began the 10-year search for a way to get off the blue pills.

Thalidomide created physical cripples; tranquillizers have been responsible for emotional cripples. I had been on Ativan two years when I began to attend psychotherapy, hoping that this would help me to come off the pills. In fact, not only did my psychiatrist continue to prescribe Ativan, but he added Tranxene to my diet and gave me weekly shots of Ritalin for therapeutic purposes. I began to look forward to these Ritalin sessions for the incredible high this drug produced. Not one of the many doctors I visited during the next 10 years would agree that I was suffering from a serious physical addiction, although I knew that this was the case. The attitude of the medical profession was that I was a weak-willed hysterical woman who leaned on tranquillizers. I became drug-riddled and I had totally lost my confidence.

One thing that I had become aware of was that withdrawal from tranquillizers was likely to be worse than coming off heroin and to take a very long time. I just couldn't see any way out of my dilemma. I thought about turning myself into a detoxification clinic, but the dangers were too great. Inadequate knowledge on behalf of the medical profession regarding the psychological trauma was an unknown factor; and anyway, the methods of detox involved other drugs and the possibility of further addiction. It was also a practical and financial impossibility to take time off from my children and my work.

I was in a constant state of semi-withdrawal, feeling ill, headachy, nauseous and weak and tense by turns and prone to violent outbursts of temper. As the years went by, my attempts to come off the pills became more and more serious. At one point I was down to 0.5 mg per day. I was working as an assistant editor at the BBC and began to go into a kind of spasm that started in my neck, and worked through my body and I was shaking violently. I was ferried home in a taxi and fell on to the street outside my house gasping and calling for help. My hands and feet were going blue, I had sharp pains in my chest and my mouth had gone numb. I was terrified as I had no idea what was happening and when I was bundled into an ambulance, the ambulance man sneered 'hysterical woman' at me. When I arrived in casualty I was rigid. The doctor who attended me was quite simply furious with me for attempting to come off the pills and made me swallow one then and there and told me to go home. My next attempt was even more disastrous. I was absolutely determined to get off the pills once and for all. I was down to 0.5 mg a day again and on that fateful night I decided to stay up and do housework until I dropped, feeling sure that the best way to cope with withdrawal would be to keep going physically. By five in the morning I was writhing with withdrawal symptoms and had to beg my husband to give me my pills back.

I could never have undergone withdrawal without NET because of the short span of time that it has taken. The actual experience of withdrawal is one of self-discovery and rebirth. Rebirth is an excruciatingly painful business. One's sense of awareness is increased to what initially seems to be an unbearable degree. I needed constant companionship during the month following the treatment. The psychological experience is that of an extended acid trip which is pretty frightening if one feels stuck in it for quite a few weeks. Without NET it could have taken a couple of years and my life would have without a doubt been totally ruined.

Going in for NET was the biggest challenge I've ever had to face. I had spoken to only one other person who had been through it and convinced me that it worked.

I was admitted to a clinic at three in the afternoon. Until this point I had only spoken to Meg Patterson on the phone. When she came into my room that afternoon I was impressed by her frail beauty but reassured by the impish glint in her eye. Her son Lorne attached the electrodes to my head. I was now linked up to the 'black box'! I turfed out my handbag and handed over every crumb of Ativan to Lorne who without a murmur washed the lot down the basin. These were the pills that had been my prison for the past 10 years.

I was in the clinic for 10 days. The withdrawal that I went through was probably physically 50 per cent less traumatic than if I had gone 'cold turkey' – a friend of mine described it accurately as 'luke-warm turkey'. Lorne was with me constantly by day, and at night I had a nurse in case of convulsions. But thanks to the 'black box' there were no convulsions.

> Without NET I would never have been able to make it through the physical withdrawal and feel that the weeks of delirium that was to follow was worth it – I earned my life back.

And five months later she wrote:

> I'm fighting fit and put on a stone since I was in the clinic! I sleep like a top these days and seem to be calm and steady . . .
>
> It's truly amazing after 10 years of 'blur' to have my memory back and all of my five senses in tip-top working order. People are constantly struck by my sense of optimism these days and my sense of purpose – not much seems to shake me – I feel like an old warrior!

Chapter 1
What is addiction?

Addiction – a diverse phenomenon

Addiction is a mystery. Nobody really knows what causes addiction, but nearly all of us will be a victim in some form at some time in our lives. Addiction is now recognized officially as one of the world's greatest social problems – possibly affecting as many people as the common cold. Although we never mind admitting to having a cold, very few of us are prepared to admit to being an addict.

Besides addictions caused by the use of illegal drugs such as heroin, cocaine and hashish, and the abuse of prescription drugs such as tranquillizers, amphetamines and sedatives, other addictive substances and habits abound. Alcohol and cigarettes will come at the top of many people's list.

Then there are the millions of tea and coffee addicts; those who need eight or more cups a day for 'more rapid and clearer flow of thought, to allay drowsiness, to increase motor activity, or to produce a keener appreciation of sensory stimuli', as one medical definition states. When withdrawn, tea and coffee were also found to produce the symptoms of addiction: 'fits of agitation, depression, loss of colour, haggard appearance, loss of appetite, heart palpitation and irregularity'. In a U S government laboratory experiment with caffeine, the addictive ingredient of tea and coffee, the offspring of rats which were fed the equivalent of 12 to 24 cups of coffee daily had an unusually high proportion of missing or deformed toes; there was even some delay in skeletal development in the offspring of rats fed the equivalent of two cups of coffee daily.

Nor does this exhaust the list of the addicted. There are workaholics who dare not stop working because of the psychological and physiological consequences; there are the gamblers who bet on horses, cards, bingo, slot machines; there are compulsive eaters, television viewers (one study showed the usual withdrawal symptoms during 30 days of TV abstinence); there are video-game players and all varieties of cult adherents.

In Britain the popular newspapers, troubled with dropping circulations, introduced 'newspaper bingo' in the early 1980s and the results were 'phenomenal' according to a report in the London *Observer*, 'putting on sales at the rate of 100,000 a month'. It continued: 'Bingo is not only a national habit, it has addictive properties, and once people are involved in a game they tend to persist to the end.'

Addiction is a more serious problem than most illnesses: it is a destructive monomania for those seeking cures for the emptiness and meaninglessness of the twentieth century.

CIGARETTES

Cigarette smoking is the most widespread example of substance abuse because, simply, nicotine reinforces and strengthens the desire to smoke and causes the users to keep on smoking. In Britain there are reported to be over 17 million nicotine addicts, on the basis that a nicotine addict is one who has tried three times to give up smoking and has failed.

> Judy, 50 years of age, had smoked 30 cigarettes daily for 30 years. She had tried repeatedly to stop smoking by many methods, including hypnosis and 'de-programming', but this only resulted in her becoming, in her own words 'a hysterical, raving lunatic'. Immediately she was put on NET her cigarettes were stopped, and throughout the five-day treatment she was completely calm and relaxed, and slept well.

A survey conducted by National Opinion Poll (NOP) showed that 42 per cent of 18 to 24 year olds smoked in 1984 compared with 37 per cent in 1981.[18] Another survey conducted in 1980 indicated that about 43 per cent of people aged 16 or over smoked cigarettes or cigars; there was little change in this figure among the population at large in 1984.[18] And in 1983, 25 per cent of children under 16 were habitual smokers.[56] About a fifth of all men and over an eighth of all women smoke sufficiently (20-plus cigarettes a day) to classify them as heavy smokers.[304] In the United States nicotine-related diseases cost $5 to $8 billion a year, not to mention another $15 million due to lost wages and productivity, and in Britain for the year 1983 it was estimated to be £1,600 million.[234]

ALCOHOL

Alcoholism has been described as one of the four worst health hazards affecting people in the western world, the other three being heart disease, cancer and mental illness. In Britain admissions to hospitals of alcohol-related problems have increased 20-fold in the past 20 years up to 1985. In the United States alcohol-related problems cost $25 billion a year. In the Soviet Union almost 60 per cent of the workforce suffers some form of alcoholism. In Venezuela about two-thirds of road casualties are caused by alcohol.

The magnitude of the alcoholism problem in Britain is only just beginning to be realized. Personal, professional and social attitudes toward the condition are so bedevilled by prejudices and traditions that it is difficult to find out what constitutes an alcoholic and how many there may be in the country. The usually quoted figure of 500,000 is derived from Jellinek's (1951) ingenious formula based on the relationship between alcoholism and cirrhosis of the liver. On this basis it has been assumed that the incidence of alcoholism among adults in Britain is about 2 to 3 per cent, with men outnumbering women in the ratio of 2:1 to 3:1, and with the proportions steadily increasing every year.

> Nancy was a 51-year-old alcoholic who arrived at the clinic in a state of extreme intoxication. In addition to four bottles of sherry daily for one and a half years, she had been taking eight yellow (5 mg) tablets of Valium daily for five years, three capsules of 25 mg of Sinequan (doxepin, a tricyclic anti-depressant) daily for nine months, and three capsules of 25 mg of Anafranil (clomipramine, a tricyclic anti-depressant) nightly for nine months. Despite this huge alcohol habit, she had neither delirium tremens (a special form of delirium, with terrifying delusions, to which drinkers are liable), nor 'the shakes'. The alcohol craving disappeared on the third day of NET and both her appearance and behaviour changed dramatically before discharge six weeks later.

According to a *Which?* magazine report in October 1984, in the past 20 years the amount of wine-drinking in Britain has more than trebled, consumption of spirits has doubled and of beer has risen by a quarter. 'Deaths from cirrhosis are sharply increasing; and much more dangerous – a third of drivers killed in car crashes, and even a quarter of pedestrians killed in road accidents, were drunk at the time of death.'[91]

The true seriousness of the problem of addictions in general, and alcoholism in particular, lies in the well-known fact that doctors themselves as a group are either the leading or near-leading victims of the condition. The situation may not be so bad as in the eighteenth century, when it was said that it was as difficult to find a sober doctor as an honest lawyer, but it is now being recognized as a serious problem.

An article in the *British Journal on Alcohol and Alcoholism* declared:

> There is considerable evidence to suggest that doctors constitute a high-risk group in respect of drinking problems. The problem of the medical practitioner who drinks excessive amounts of alcohol has still received remarkably little attention by the profession or the public. The view that alcoholism is a particular hazard for doctors is supported by the fact that the liver cirrhosis mortality rate in England and Wales for doctors is known to be 3.5 times that among the general population. On this basis Dr Max Glatt has estimated that there are 2,000 to 3,000 alcoholic doctors in the country at present.
>
> In addition, there may be a large number of medical practitioners whose professional performance is impaired by alcoholic excess. In a clinical area of this magnitude where concealment is a common attitude it is impossible to 'count heads' accurately...
>
> George Orwell observed, 'A known fact may be so unbearable that it is habitually pushed aside and not allowed to enter logical processes.'[229] Doctors with an alcohol problem may find acceptance of this problem quite unbearable. Moreover, relatives, friends and colleagues often enter into a process of concealment or 'cover-up' which may be motivated by fear of endangering their respectable image in the community and profession.
>
> It may be feared too that revelation of the problem will lead to enforced withdrawal from professional employment, undesired stigma resulting from referral to psychiatry, loss of income or superannuation, and perhaps sacrifice of goodwill and promotion. The willingness of the individual and his colleagues to confront the issue of alcoholism in a professional man or woman more often than not arises out of kindness or loyalty, from embarrassment; it is hoped, usually quite unrealistically, that if the problem is ignored, it will go away.[282]

This was written about doctors, but it can be equally applied to other professions. Estimates indicate that alcoholism alone costs

British industry at least £500 million a year - and that is based on statistics which are admitted to be conservative. Company directors have been known to state that their firm has no problems with alcoholism in management, when it has been widely known that several of their own directors and managers are alcoholics. At the workforce level, at least 5 per cent are suffering from alcoholism, with approximately a third in the later stages. That means the Civil Service could have over 10,000 alcoholics, and any company with 20,000 employees could have about 1,000 alcoholics. It has also been estimated that at least four-fifths of alcoholics go undetected at their work-place.[216] In a general practice of 3,000 patients in a densely populated, urbanized, mainly working-class population there are possibly 30 heavy drinkers, 27 problem drinkers and 25 alcoholics.

When the official figure of alcoholics for Britain was said to be a half-million (1976) it was estimated that 150,000 were women. However, these figures were qualified by the observation that there were probably another four million affected indirectly by alcoholism or excessive drinking and that is not including the families and friends of alcoholics.

The alcohol problem relating to children was 50 times greater than the drug problem, 50 per cent of boys and 30 per cent of girls between 13 and 15 drinking alcohol on 'a fairly regular basis'.[8] The same report stated that women go from controlled to uncontrolled drinking in as short a time as three years, compared with the usual time of eight to twelve for men. And 'current research ... has revealed evidence that even moderate amounts of alcohol intake associated with "social drinking" can result in mild cognitive impairments.'[249]

Stress - causing drug misuse

The problem of alcoholism in recent years has been further complicated by the increasing tendency to use other chemical substances at the same time. It is rare nowadays to find an alcoholic who uses no other drugs, even if it is only sleeping pills.

Alcoholism in Britain is 20 times as prevalent as so-called 'hard-drug' dependence. But when so-called 'soft-drugs' - barbiturates, tranquillizers, amphetamines, nicotine - are included then the proportions are reversed. To them may be added the analgesic addicts with their overuse or misuse of drugs like aspirin or paracetamol. When these two are mixed with codeine or caffeine to induce mood-alteration, or for stress or insomnia, they can be as habit-forming as the hard drugs.

Dr Sidney Cohen of the University of California writes of barbiturates (all other sleeping pills have similar effects): 'Over days or weeks tolerance evolves, requiring either increasing amounts of the soporific or a loss of its efficacy.' When they are stopped, the result is 'REM rebound with its nightmarish, sleep-disturbing dreams. Patients then demand re-institution of their sleeping.'[62]

> Sam was 24 and a heroin addict. He had smoked or snorted about 2 grams daily for four years, as well as a gram or more of cocaine daily for 11 years (he had a large hole in his nasal septum from this habit); every day for six months he had taken 5,000 milligrams (50 capsules) of the barbiturate Tuinal, and 20 tablets of paracetamol. The paracetamol was for the excruciating headaches which had developed from his excessive drug abuse. Because these headaches were so severe I sent him to be investigated for a possible brain tumour, but none was found. On his admission I stopped all drugs immediately, and except for one brief convulsion of a few seconds' duration on the fifth day of treatment he had no further trouble. All headaches had disappeared by the time he was discharged three weeks later.

The problem of stress, and its solution, accounts for the largest financial investment in research by the wealthiest pharmaceutical companies in the world. The importance of stress in a variety of illnesses has been described by Dr Hans Selye (see p. 151).

A report from the authoritative Institute for the Study of Drug Dependence Library and Information Service states:

> One such study in 1977 suggested that 12 per cent of the adult population in England and Wales had taken a prescribed psychotropic drug in the previous fortnight, and that some 7 per cent had first been prescribed that drug a year or more ago. An earlier (1971) study found that 1 in 7 of the adult UK population had taken a tranquillizer or sedative in the past year, and that over 8 per cent of the population had been taking them every day for at least a month.[304]

The report continues:

> The proportion of women making short- or long-term use of prescribed psychotropics is double the proportion of men. There is evidence from a Marplan survey that a third of all women have at

> some time been prescribed tranquillizers, over a quarter sleeping pills, and that very nearly half (46 per cent) of the women in Britain have been prescribed one or the other at some time in their life. This same survey found that about a fifth of the women ever prescribed these drugs were taking them at least three times a week...
>
> There is some research evidence that 15 to 20 per cent of patients prescribed sleeping pills become dependent on the drug and that tranquillizers lose their therapeutic value and effectiveness after four months consecutive use.[65]

To compound the disaster of this situation, a representative sample from an inner city general practice, studied for three years and reported in 1984, showed that 44 per cent of the prescriptions written for psychotropic drugs were repeat prescriptions written without a consultation.[158]

The same ISDD report concludes that some 5 million people in Britain have taken cannabis, at some time, with at least a million taking the drug in a year. Nearly 1.3 million used amphetamines (in 1973) and 650,000 had used LSD.

MARIJUANA

Marijuana ('grass') or cannabis ('hash') are claimed by users to be less harmful than alcohol and other drugs of abuse – including cigarettes – and there seems little doubt that this is true. Nevertheless, many heroin addicts say that they would probably never have taken heroin had they not first experienced the mind-altering effects of marijuana or hashish. Most habitual users also admit that regular 'smoking' diminishes their drive and motivation and many know they are addicted to it because they are unable to stop their daily use. Relatively few request help to stop using it because, they say, 'it is surely better to smoke than to get drunk every evening'.

But eventually, a considerable number will experience serious problems. Medical journals are reporting an increasing number of psychoses resulting from use of marijuana or cannabis alone.[41, 50, 307]

> James, 35, came from a family of alcoholics and had himself been drinking excessively since his teens. He had been taken off alcohol repeatedly but was always given substitute drugs which made him unable to function normally. Finally, he managed to stop both drugs and alcohol but only by substituting 7 to 15 joints of marijuana daily, along with about 10 cups of coffee as a 'speedball' addiction. Without these he was unable to cope with his anxiety and depression.

> Ten days of NET with no marijuana and no coffee made him feel able to cope with problems accumulated over about 20 years.

A high proportion of users also report short-term adverse effects from marijuana: fearfulness, confusion, excessive dependency, intense aggressive impulses, panic, paranoid reactions, hallucinations and distortions of body image. However, these occur more frequently in first-time users than in regular users.[222]

In a perceptive survey into the non-therapeutic use of psychoactive drugs in the US in 1983, Dr Armand Nicholi of Harvard Medical School says it has 'spread with explosive force into an epidemic of extraordinary scope involving all regions of the country, all socioeconomic classes and all age groups ... Marijuana is the most widely used illicit drug; one quarter of the entire US population have used the drug and 20 million people use it daily.'[222] It is reported that 5 million now use it in Britain.[107]

TRANQUILLIZERS AND SEDATIVES

An investigation commissioned by the Department of Health and Social Security in 1982 into ways of monitoring drug abuse, quotes one of the research team as saying:

> If I were a G.P. the area that would concern me more than heroin would be the benzodiazepines. There is a massive area of semi-abuse of drugs mixed with alcohol by a huge range of people who do not fit into the stereotype of the drug addict at all. Among them are mothers who discover the effects of a drug like Valium when taken with strong lager in 'Valium-Special Brew afternoons' ... The problem may not be as dramatic as heroin addiction, but it is of as much concern.

Physicians report 'Prolonged use of these drugs produce many unpleasant symptoms such as loss of concentration and memory, decline in psychomotor performance (thus leading to accidents at work and while driving), depression and emotional anaesthesia.'[268] But even after a single small dose (2.5 mg) of lorazepam given to healthy volunteers, a 1984 study at the University of London reported that 'subjects were unimpaired in the recall of material presented before drug treatment, but were severely impaired if presentation was after drug administration, irrespective of whether learning was tested by recognition or recall'.[192] Rats on benzodiazepines sometimes lose their coping mechanisms for a very long time after withdrawal, and the same appears to be true for humans.[319]

> Johnny, 30, had been an alcoholic for 10 years, but only on weekends because, during the week, his job required skill and concentration. For eight years he had been taking up to 100 milligrams of Valium daily (10 blue or 20 yellow tablets), legally prescribed by his doctor, for his bouts of 'depression'. On Valium he was increasingly losing control, was anxious, bad-tempered, dysphoric. When he tried to stop the Valium by himself he felt a paralysing sense of 'plunging into a bottomless pit'. With NET he came off both alcohol and Valium easily, with no convulsions, and only one night of poor sleep. Ten months later he wrote: 'I cannot say how grateful we all are for my treatment. It unveiled an unknown quality in myself of loving and caring for my family.'

A recent *British Medical Journal* editorial[322] states that 'several investigations have shown quite unequivocally that benzodiazepines' such as Valium, Librium, Ativan, Serenid-D, 'may produce pharmacological dependence in therapeutic dosage even after only 6 weeks of regular use', although 'more than half can stop treatment without any important withdrawal symptoms'. Tyrer, an expert in this field, comments that 'the finding that 44 per cent of patients taking long-term diazepam had withdrawal symptoms despite gradual reduction in medication is disturbing'. The patients referred to had been taking Valium 5 to 20 mg daily for at least three months and the dosage was reduced in a stepwise fashion over a period of three months.[323]

A 1985 Scottish double-blind study has confirmed that 'diazepam (Valium) can produce rebound anxiety and withdrawal symptoms when used in moderate doses and for what has previously been regarded as a safe length of time' (6 weeks).[252] (For details of withdrawal symptomatology from various drugs, see Appendix III.)

Unfortunately, when a patient on a tranquillizer stops or reduces the drug and develops withdrawal symptoms, anxiety in particular, both patient and doctor tend to mistake this for a return of the pre-existing anxiety instead of the real cause, drug-withdrawal; the doctor is likely to either increase the dosage or prescribe an additional drug.

Such symptoms may develop even while the patient is still taking the drug because of development of tolerance to the given dosage, and the established fact that such drugs are ineffective in the treatment of anxiety after four months' continuous use.[65] (See Susan's story in the Introduction.) In fact, clinical trials have shown that 'when given to patients with low anxiety levels benzodiazepines have been found to be no better than placebo'.[51]

An ISSD report states: 'There is widespread suspicion that numbers running into the 100,000s may be dependent on sedatives or tranquillizers prescribed by their doctors.'[264] This refers to ' "respectable", law-abiding people' over and above the drug-abusers who in the late-1970s and 1980s are mostly polydrug users. A recent MORI poll claimed that 1.5 million people in Britain are presently dependent on benzodiazepines.

My own survey of 88 consecutive admissions in 1980 for treatment showed that the average number of different drugs used by each drug or alcohol addict since the start of the abuse was 19.8. The number of drugs being actively abused at the time of admission was three drugs per person[242] - and polydrug use has a worse prognosis than single drug abuse.[62] For 186 admissions, 30 per cent were regularly taking a tranquillizer (usually Valium) in addition to other drugs or alcohol.

Until recent changes were introduced, the National Health Service needed some £20 million to pay for the 50 million annual prescriptions for anti-anxiety drugs and tranquillizers.

COCAINE

Another popular combination is the mixture of heroin and cocaine, mostly in order to prolong the 'high' of the cocaine and to offset the sudden drop into cocaine depression. Dr David Smith, the founder and medical director of the Haight Ashbury Medical Clinic in San Francisco, said recently that increasing numbers of American middle-class cocaine users are now mixing it with heroin to modify the stimulant effects of cocaine - whether the cocaine is taken by sniffing, injection or free-basing. He also stated categorically that despite the claims of some researchers in earlier years, cocaine had now emerged as 'the most addictive drug' in popular use. Many of my patients would support this claim, but it appears that not all who try it become addicted.

Time magazine reported in 1981 that 'if all the international dealers who supply the United States cocaine market - not even including the retailers – were to form a single corporation, it would probably rank seventh on the *Fortune* 500 list top companies, between the Ford Company ($37 billion in revenue) and Gulf Oil Corporation ($26.5 billion)'.[87]

In 1983 *Time* said that:

> Among the 4 million to 5 million Americans who regularly use cocaine, drug counsellors estimate that 5 per cent to 20 per cent – at least 200,000, perhaps 1 million – are now profoundly dependent on cocaine, a new corps as numerous as heroin addicts. During the past two years or so, the number of Americans who have used the drug climbed from 15 million to 20 million and is rising still: every day some 5,000 neophytes sniff a line of coke for the first time. Cocaine has become a $25 billion business, about three times as big as the recording and movie industries put together. Selling coke is, in the words of one US drug official, 'the most lucrative of all under-world ventures'.[11]

In 1984, cocaine, marijuana and heroin in the USA was a business worth $80 billion a year.[75] In Britain, the fastest growing drug of abuse is cocaine.[107] Only 26.65 lbs were seized by Customs and Excise in 1982, but 156.37 lbs were seized in 1983.[92]

As recently as the late-1970s Britain was just a staging-post in the international drug trafficking system, but it is now a centre and market in its own right, together with Holland, France and West Germany. The increasing popularity and demand for cocaine in social circles in Britain provides an attractive market for the well-organized criminal syndicates with an already existing distribution system, beyond the capacity of the official law-enforcement agencies to combat.

Since the mid-1970s, cocaine has become the wealthy person's choice of 'recreational drug' in Britain and is often passed around the table at the end of dinner, as port used to be. Its current price is £55.70 per gram, or teaspoonful (typically 30 per cent to 70 per cent pure), and the average amount taken by a regular user is 1 to 2 grams daily. 'Free-basing' of cocaine, a more expensive method than sniffing but giving a more rapid and more intense effect, does not yet appear to be as popular in Britain as it is in the USA.

The reasons for the attraction of cocaine have been well described in a 1984 article in the *International Journal of the Addictions*:

> Cocaine is a seductive and intensely coercive drug, one of the most powerful pharmacological reinforcers known ... It reduces anxiety and heightens the distinctiveness of the ego, making the user feel more aggressive, optimistic, and self-assured. Heavy ... use of cocaine ... produces an experience so close to completeness that the user feels compelled to return again and again, hoping that the ultimate consummation will occur. [But it never does.] The heavy user tolerates the adverse effects of cocaine because the drug briefly lifts him out of depression, helps ward off the Shadow, and seems to promise fulfilment of a need for balance and unity.[293]

> Archie, at 35, had been on cocaine for 14 years, gradually increasing his habit to 5 grams daily at the time of admission to the clinic. He had also snorted 1 gram of heroin daily for 10 years. He was terrified at the possibility of having no cocaine, for he had not been without it for a single day in two years. Six months after successful detoxification and discharge from NET treatment he told a gathering of doctors at a medical conference that NET had not only freed him from addiction but had brought about an actual change for the better in his character.

As with cannabis, there must be many 'recreational' users of cocaine who do not become addicted, but it is impossible to foretell who will fall victim. Most addicts who have requested treatment have said, 'In the early days I was quite sure that I would be different from the others – that I would be able to keep it under control and not become addicted.'

A typical story is that the young business executive or professional individual becomes so up-tight with cocaine that he 'mellows' it with a spot of heroin (his friends assure him that he will not become addicted to heroin if he uses it in this way) but, inevitably, he does, and the downward slide accelerates. The situation was recently highlighted by Mark Gold of New York, who with some colleagues set up a national helpline in 1983 for cocaine users. They have received up to 1,000 calls a day (over 70,000 in the first three months) and obtained a 30-minute interview, with their consent, for a random sample of 306 intranasal cocaine users. They report:

> Most were white (85%) and employed (77%). 37% were earning over $25,000 per year. They had been using cocaine for an average of 4 years. Current use averaged 4.5 g per week at a cost of over $450 per week. 65% reported using tranquillizers, alcohol, or heroin to counteract the overstimulation or rebound dysphoria ('crash') after

> cocaine use. *Over 50% of these intranasal cocaine users said they felt addicted to cocaine*, could not refuse cocaine when it was available, found themselves unable to stop for at least one month, experienced significant distress without cocaine, and had withdrawal symptoms of marked depression, and anergy when they tried to stop using the drug. [my italics]
>
> 36% reported dealing in cocaine and 20% were stealing from work, family, or friends to support their cocaine habit. Over 90% reported adverse ... consequences, including: chronic fatigue (74%), insomnia (81%), nosebleeds (54%), headaches (58%), loss of sex drive (41%), depression (75%), irritability (78%), memory/concentration problems (61%), paranoia (58%), impaired job functioning (34%), impaired relationships (59%), and depletion of all finances (34%). Cocaine-related suicide attempts (8%), automobile accidents (8%), and brain seizures with loss of consciousness (8%) were also reported.[335]

Their later findings show that:

> In adolescents cocaine abuse seems to lead to more rapid and more severe drug-related consequences than it does in adults. The time lapse between first use of cocaine and the onset of deteriorated functioning averaged 4 years in the adult compared with 1.5 years in the adolescent. Moreover, the adolescents reported a higher frequency of cocaine-related brain seizures, automobile accidents, suicide attempts, and violent behaviour.[336]

Cocaine erodes the nasal septum and many who take the drug by sniffing suffer unpleasant symptoms from this. Sensitivity to the drug or an overdose can cause collapse, convulsions and death.[343]

STIMULANTS AND HALLUCINOGENS

Occasionally, doctors actually prescribe amphetamine-like drugs or other appetite suppressants to girls who want to slim for reasons of inferiority or vanity or sport, and so start the addictive process. Fortunately, more doctors are now aware of this problem. Continued use of the stimulant amphetamines, widely available on the illicit market - used by students to help them stay awake while studying, or by athletes to reduce fatigue (as a cheap form of cocaine) - may produce irritability and apprehension, even in low doses. Frequent large doses may produce brain damage, repetitive grinding of the teeth, and psychosis or paranoia.[222]

The Department of Education and Science has estimated that up to 10 per cent of British children between the ages of 12 and 17 have experimented with glue-sniffing.[107] Although the sniffing of glue or other inhalants, or use of psychedelics, may occasionally cause paranoia or death (roughly 80 deaths each year in the UK are associated with solvent abuse[76]), there is no evidence for physical or psychological dependence. In fact, most of my patients say they used LSD for about a year and then stopped it without any problem. Some claim the LSD gives psychological and even spiritual insights, but I have yet to meet anyone who showed either intellectual or behavioural evidence of any value obtained through LSD experiences (see Koestler's comments, page 189).

Inhalants, of course, cause only harmful effects. PCP (phencyclidine, known as 'angel dust') is frequently associated with extreme violence and paranoid behaviour; probably many deaths result from behavioural toxicity caused by this drug,[222] particularly with the disturbing trend, detected in 1983 in USA, towards intravenous PCP use.[218]

HEROIN

The figures for heroin imports into Britain are even more staggering than those for cocaine. It is officially reported in 1984 that £6 million-worth of heroin is coming into the country through Dover and Heathrow alone *every week*.[136] Customs officials comment, 'We're a laughing stock. We know there's smuggling going on but just haven't got the staff to deal with it ... We must be missing 90% of the drugs smuggled into this country.'[248]

The majority of drug addicts start their period of addiction by taking marijuana (by mouth in 'chocolate cookies' or smoking it mixed with tobacco and rolled to form a 'joint') or shandy or a wide variety of pills. Often, youngsters do not even know what is in the pills. They even try out 'skag', not realizing it is heroin. In the past few years, unemployed teenagers have been going straight to 'skag' (a 'bag' costs about £5) because it is so cheap and so easy to get. They have no hope of getting work – no hope for anything. Heroin gives them an illusion of transcendence in a despairing situation.

Heroin is the most addictive of all 'recreational' drugs because of its powerful euphoria. A Hong Kong addict, expressed it succinctly, in a film made by my husband, Adrian Cowell and Chris Menges, called 'The Opium Trail', when he said 'How can you fight a dream?'

The majority use it intravenously ('mainlining') in order to get a greater effect from a smaller amount of the drug. However, all other ways of using it are *equally* addictive - snorting (sniffing it through the nose, usually through a rolled up bank-note or a special metal tube, sometimes gold), or 'chasing the dragon', a method that used to be confined to the Far East but is now increasingly popular in Britain (the heroin is placed on a piece of foil, a match or cigarette-lighter held under the foil to vaporize the heroin, and the vapour inhaled through a roll of paper).

Street heroin in 1984 cost £50-£60 per gram (typically 30-60 per cent pure), whereas two years previously it was £120 per gram (a common *daily* amount used by middle class or criminal addicts). Young addicts now say 'it is as easy to buy heroin as it is to buy a bag of sugar' and the proportion of young teenagers using it is increasing horrendously. A 10-year-old addict was reported recently. To sustain their costly habit, they are driven to crime, prostitution or drug-dealing. And it is not the drug-dealers who recruit new addicts: it is the addicts themselves who do this by 'percenting', i.e. by keeping one or two packets of a quota and selling the remainder to friends.

Heroin produces an extremely powerful physical dependency in almost all who use it recreationally, although there are widely differing reports on the length of time it takes to become irreparably addicted. Some have told me that by the second dose they were 'hooked'; others claim they have used it for many months before it became a necessary part of their lives.

When 'hooked', heroin addicts can function normally for a varying length of time. They feel that their heroin dose keeps them 'normal', but tolerance inevitably develops and an increasingly larger dose is required to produce 'normality', let alone a high. Eventually, not even a high can be achieved, and the abuse is continued only because of the withdrawal agonies experienced when the dose is not taken.

> Sarah, 22, was a registered drug addict who had been receiving 400 milligrams of pure (100 per cent) heroin daily from a government drug dependency unit. She had begun mainlining 3 g of street heroin at the age of 17, and the government heroin replaced this. Every night she took 'very large' doses of sedatives. In addition, she had taken 30 milligrams of linctus methadone daily for three years. Four hours before she was admitted for NET treatment she injected 900 milligrams of pure heroin intravenously and drank two one-pint bottles of linctus methadone. Her tolerance for drugs was so high

she didn't even fall asleep, although her speech was slurred and her eyes glazed. She had only mild discomfort during her early treatment with NET and was exercising enthusiastically within 48 hours.

Effects on family

Addicts often express bitterness and resentment against a father who drinks heavily, or a mother whose cupboard is full of Valium and sleeping pills, and both probably also hooked on cigarettes – all legalized drugs. The parents ignore the established fact that their addiction is often more lethal than their offsprings' addiction.

Reports that morphine or heroin may compromise the body's immune system are contradictory[19] and heroin is possibly still the safest psychoactive drug in existence; it is certainly less harmful than these legal drugs. But people die of heroin abuse because of deliberate or accidental overdosing, or from poisonous substances dealers have used to dilute the heroin powder, or from dirty needles which cause health-destroying or fatal infections.

It is arguable that a family suffers more by having an alcoholic parent in the home than a drug addict child. Certainly, most narcotic addicts who survive till their mid-30s seem to 'mature out' of their drug abuse without any treatment: alcohol abuse knows no age limit.

Free or even legal distribution of heroin or methadone or any other drug will only prolong the problem both for government and for the addicts themselves. Governments should provide the curative treatment needed to enable addicts to stop their drug abuse completely, because almost all of them will want to stop, sooner or later.

Chapter 2
The British scene and the inadequacies of current treatments

Statistics of drug abuse

Britain is in the throes of a drug explosion. The number of narcotic addicts known to the Home Office increased by 70 per cent between 1980 and 1982[138] and by a further 30 per cent in 1983. Sir Bernard Braine, MP, reported in the House of Commons in the spring of 1984 that 'the Home Office now knew of 10,271 addicts "but the fieldworkers tell me that that represents only about one tenth of the total."'[84] Within that total there was a 50 per cent increase of new addicts notified for the first time.[136]

In fact, many fieldworkers would agree with one researcher who claims that 'a truer figure of people abusing one or a mixture of drugs in Britain is two hundred thousand'.[107]

Scotland reported 85 notifications in 1978 and 574 in 1983 - an increase of 575 per cent. The accepted figure of 50,000 opioid addicts does not include occasional and intermittent users.[134] It is estimated that there will be about 100,000 officially recognized drug abusers in Britain in the next five years[138]; fieldworkers insist that this is still only the tip of the iceberg. The previous chapter has demonstrated the astronomical scale of the real drug problem in the country.

Europe also has had a heavy drug problem for the past decade, but the incidence is still increasing. For example, health officials in Bonn estimate that 1 million West German children aged 11 to 15 regularly take some kind of drug. In 1984, France is reported to have 120,000 addicts, Italy 250,000, with 472 drug deaths in West Germany in 1983, 190 in France and 257 in Italy.[350] The figure for heroin and opiate addicts in Europe is probably nearer to 2 million.[107]

In the USA, there are half a million known heroin addicts[309] but the true figure is much higher.[107] US government monitoring agencies have estimated conservatively that drug use in the factory

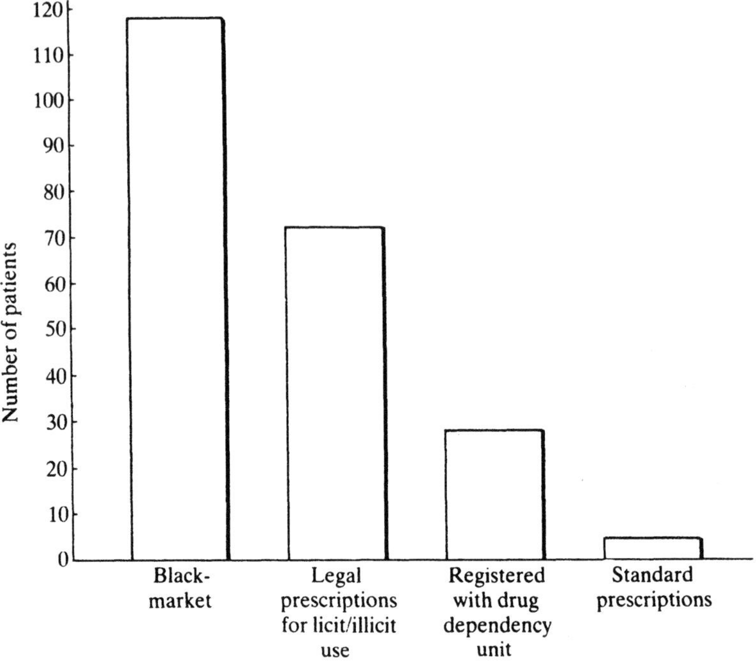

Figure 2.1 Source of drugs obtained by addicts. 'Standard prescriptions' indicate those written by doctors to meet a genuine need.

and office is costing the country $25 billion (£17.24 billion) a year.[107]

In India, where opium-smoking is a traditional, rich man's pleasure, heroin addiction has lately hit the middle classes; Delhi alone is estimated to have 90,000 heroin addicts.[182] In Pakistan in 1980 addiction was negligible; in 1984 there are more than 150,000 Pakistani addicts.[93] Malaysia reports 400,000 drug abusers.[303] The figures - and tragedies - go on escalating endlessly.

There is also the massive 'Mandrax trail' from India to South Africa. The sleeping pill Mandrax (called Quaalude in the USA) was a very popular substitute for heroin in the early 1970s, but it was particularly dangerous and was taken off the British market in 1973. It is now manufactured illegally in India and widely available in South Africa,[126] where it is the fastest-growing drug problem, particularly amongst affluent whites.[203] Recently, both Mandrax and Seconal have become a problem in China and Hong Kong.[102]

In this country, one researcher reported by *New Society* counted

272 addicts buying and selling drugs in the Haymarket in London in a six-hour period on a Saturday afternoon. This drug-trafficking is made possible by the careless overprescribing by doctors as well as through massive illegal imports from the Third World. Many doctors do not know or care that it is not difficult for an addict to get a prescription for 70 amphetamines changed into hundreds of pounds, from which he can buy his heroin or cocaine.

Among my patients, while 117 of them stated that their drug-source was the black-market, 72 claimed to be obtaining their drugs through prescriptions provided by doctors in general practice (see Figure 2.1).

Available 'treatment'

Despite a 15-fold increase in the addiction problem in Britain since I first became interested in the early 1960s, there are now fewer clinics and numbers of available beds than when I started - my own clinic had to close down in 1981 because of lack of funding, official and voluntary. Local GPs in London, certainly in the Camden and Islington area, are now treating as many opioid addicts as the local drug units, and for every opioid addict there is at least one other with severe tranquillizer/alcohol problems.

In 1977 an exasperated general practitioner wrote to the Secretary of State at the DHSS, with copies to the Home Office Ombudsmen and the Health Service Ombudsman. He asked three simple questions: who was locally responsible for the treatment of drug addicts in his area; where was there a facility; and when would one be provided. It took 18 months to get a reply.

In pursuing his investigations into why it took so long to get these apparently simple questions answered, the Ombudsman discovered a maze of misunderstanding and bureaucratic cover-up in which the patients were the only sufferers. After about two years the Ombudsman's report to the doctor admitted 'the position disclosed by my enquiry is deplorable. The story has been one of obvious delay and confusion throughout in deciding upon and providing drug dependency unit out-patient facilities.'

This incident was reported in the summer (1980) issue of *Drug Link*, the newsletter of the Institute for the Study of Drug Dependence, and it concluded:

> Addiction is a muddled moral/medical/criminal concept uneasily, and only quite recently, found a home in NHS psychiatric practice (sic). If the (Ombudsman's) Report is anything to go by, the administration of addiction treatment is every bit as muddled as the concept of addiction itself.

Government's irresponsibility

In July 1984, Sir Bernard Braine commented in the House of Commons, 'One of the most frequent complaints made to me earlier this year was that many doctors did not want to know about the problem ... There is a division in the medical profession about treatment itself.' Since 1972 I have repeatedly expressed the same conclusions, not to be provocative but out of frustration, bewilderment and, often, despair with the profession I love and to which I have dedicated my life.

Sir Bernard continued, 'On 13 April I drew the attention of the House to the appalling escalation of the drug problem ... The reality was that while the Advisory Committee on the Misuse of Drugs made over 40 recommendations as long ago as December 1982, nothing was done.'[140] In 1981, I offered my services to the Minister of Health to train medical and paramedical staff in NET techniques. He sent back a polite letter saying that central government does not employ consultants, and that I should apply to an area health authority.

Sir Bernard then described the situation as researched by the BBC 'Panorama' programme:

> 'The overall picture was one of uncertainty, ignorance and inability to cope - which, from health authorities generally reluctant to admit deficiencies in their service, can only be in itself an underestimate of the crisis.' What sort of response will the Government get from these authorities? Are they aware, even now, of the gravity of the crisis? I am beginning to doubt it.[140]

This was also my experience - polite disinterest, inept bureaucracy, deliberate neglect, total lack of official cooperation at every level unless pursued with stubborn persistence - until I had no option but to go to the United States in 1981 for over three years.

The official lack of interest is not the only barrier between the addict and the caring doctor. In addition there are the multi-million pound alcohol, tobacco and pharmaceutical vested interests, with their callous indifference to the problem and their expensive advertizing campaigns in the media, so grossly disproportionate to their willingness to spend money in the alleviation of the problem. Then behind them looms an even greater obstacle, the sinister criminal syndicates with their own multi-billion pound interests.

The media has made efforts to publicize the rapid escalation of drug abuse but there are only a few signs either of any official comprehension of the problem in Britain or of any attempts to formulate a central policy to combat it.

Central government should decide what treatment has been shown to be effective medically, cost-effective and most easily accomplished in a reasonably short time. They should then take responsibility for putting this into effect for as long as the need exists, instead of forcing area health authorities to struggle with a problem in which most of the medical and nursing personnel have had no training or experience.

Government's demonstrable reluctance to become involved appears to stem from their past experience of failure with official maintenance centres providing heroin and the even less successful methadone; and it seems that they are unable to propose a viable alternative.

Summing up the heroin situation in its winter (1982) issue, the ISDD *Drug Link* information letter states:

> Pulling the strands together, the prospects for heroin in Britain in the 1980s are being marked by:
>
> 1 Large parts of the population, and in particular the part caught in the unemployment limbo between school and work, predisposed towards the exploitation of an effective anxiety tension reducer, euphoriant, and money spinner - and here heroin's combination of pharmacological and financial assets fits the bill to a tee.
>
> 2 A heroin supply 'system' capable of increasing the quantity delivered and reducing its price without reducing the quality, and capable of adapting to political and military disruptions without significantly interrupting the flow.
>
> 3 And perhaps largely created by this supply, increasing numbers of people seemingly financially able and psychologically willing to obtain and use the heroin on offer.

Despite the monumental scale of the drug problem, despite the lip-service paid by governments and medical groups to the seriousness of the problem, despite the fact that both of those groups admit that, to their knowledge, there is no promising cure for the treatment of addictions on the horizon, I received from them only polite and professional expressions of interest - and no financial aid. The media, although they had their own vested interest in pursuing the bizarre and the sensational, have discharged their responsibility to the public with regard to my work with serious and balanced presentations since 1973. So the professional politicians in governments and medical establishments are without excuse in their reluctance - or even neglect - to pursue relevant investigations.

In 1983 the government offered £6 million, spread over only three years, for drug services in England, available to local authorities or voluntary bodies. According to the spring (1984) issue of *Drug Link*, 'many local authorities baulked at the prospect of redirecting local effort towards drug-takers and, inevitably, away from other needy groups'. They report that 'in this time of financial constraints, without security as to future funding arrangements, it is unlikely that many additional services would be established', and that 'the problem in this field is where money should come from once the pump is primed'. The possibility of permanent, central funding has been rejected.[262]

In a parliamentary debate on 13 July 1984,[138] it was claimed that 50 per cent of young people aged between 14 and 25 years on Merseyside regularly use heroin (confirmed by the Merseyside drugs council[141]), and that 'the country was confronted with a plague. The picture was one of all ages and all social classes being involved. It was a terrifying problem. Large areas of the country had no medical treatment facilities and many people did not seek help.' Government has announced that it will give an extra £1 million to improve services, an amount denounced by Labour MPs as 'derisory'; they claimed that '*£20 million a year* was needed to cope with Britain's rising crisis of drug addiction' (my italics). The other side of the coin is 'the dearth of trained personnel interested in drug abuse'[262]. Out of allocation of funds for 1984, only one new residential facility of any kind is to be established, and that by a voluntary body.[251]

At the British Medical Association's annual meeting on 5 July 1984, one speaker stated that 'a third of secondary school pupils had experimented with drugs or solvents'; recent school-leavers whom I have questioned consider 50 to 60 per cent to be a more realistic figure. Another speaker said that:

> For the first time in this country, there is no such place as a drug-free environment. The greatest problem in treating addicts is that heroin is now so much cheaper and so easy to obtain ... Addicts were becoming younger and younger. Sixteen and seventeen year-olds were dependent on heroin. Sniffing heroin seemed more addictive than injecting it ... A week's regular use and you are hooked. They spend most of their dole money on heroin, and beg, borrow and steal and in the case of girls turn to prostitution to pay for their habit. Of these people up to one third are likely to die.[315]

The Government Advisory Council on the Misuse of Drugs issued a report in July 1984, concluding that 'present services for drug misusers ... are now less able than ever to cope with the problems of drug misuse'[253]. To quote the 13 July 1984 parliamentary debate again:

> There are 50,000 to 60,000 addicts ... The figures showing the latest big increase have not even appeared yet ... To face that level ... NHS outpatient capacity for drug treatment in the whole country totals 2,000. Even the clinics that provide that service are characterized by staff shortages, the freezing of vacancies and lack of continuity. That means that only from 1,000 to as few as 600 people can make use of those 2,000 national places ... The NHS inpatient capacity to cope with the problem is at the princely total of about 110 beds, and many of them are used for those suffering from alcohol addiction.[142]

But there is little point in increasing beds or outpatient services if there is no central policy of treatment, the existing methods having been demonstrably inadequate. The few existing drug rehabilitation centres and therapeutic communities are booked solidly in advance for several months (since each resident is expected to stay for 12 to 18 months). Few churches seem to be concerned, and those that are concerned are not equipped to provide the informed and structured counselling necessary for drug addicts and alcoholics. There are voluntary organizations for marriage guidance, for potential suicides, and for family counselling, but none of them have personnel trained to cope with drug addicts and alcoholics in a specialized 'recovery programme'.

Some of this is now being said publicly in Parliament.

> If we are to attach the kind of priority that the Government say they attach to dealing with the treatment of those who misuse drugs, there needs to be a system of *central* Government funding, *tied to the delivery of specific facilities and projects.* That is the only way to ensure that there is a national and comprehensive system of treatment and after-care for drug addicts. The ad hoc pump-priming mechanisms in which the Government are involving themselves will in no way deal with the long-term problem with which we are confronted.[139] (my italics)

Methadone maintenance

The official reluctance to underwrite any realistic efforts to tackle the scale of the drug explosion is exacerbated by the tragic waste of resources which are channelled towards ineffective 'cures'.

Millions of dollars have been spent in the USA in recent years trying to find a substitute drug for heroin. A 1981 USA figure states that some 80,000 heroin-dependent people were being given the substitute drug methadone in about 800 methadone maintenance clinics.[62] The 31 drug dependence units in Britain (DDUs) who treat registered addicts on an outpatient basis, at first supplied heroin and cocaine free in the late-1960s, now give no cocaine, although a few still supply heroin, and most new patients receive oral or injectable methadone (Physeptone) with, sometimes, antidepressants, anxiolytics or sleeping pills in addition.

Dr Stanton Peele, a psychologist from Columbia University and author of the well-known book *Love and Addiction* writes:

> The many mistaken and costly ideas about defeating addiction that have been propagated all stem from the same fundamental error. This is the failure to understand that a person is addicted to an experience. If a cure for addiction fails to take into account a person's need for the addictive experience, he or she will simply be set loose to seek a comparable experience elsewhere.[243]

Dr Peele continues: 'Methadone maintenance is one example of this wrong-headed approach to combating addiction ... Yet its founders, Drs Dole and Nyswander, note that methadone maintenance's impact has been minimal "at best"[89].'

This is clearly illustrated by a letter I received in 1984.

Currently I am taking 50 milligrams daily of methadone. I've been on a maintenance program in New York for the last four years. Before that I was using heroin and other narcotics (dilaudid, demerol) for several years. Although methadone has allowed me to clean up my lifestyle so that I am now working full time, it has also caused changes in my body and mind and I want to be free of my addiction to it.

I've become lethargic, I've gained 30 lbs., and where I was once vivacious and outgoing, I am now quiet and withdrawn. I seem to have lost my ambition and drive, and I lack the physical stamina to really enjoy life. And the sad part is that I never feel quite normal. I feel sick without the methadone yet I feel sick with it too, I feel always drugged, artificial, absent minded.

I started on methadone because I couldn't stand the pain and anxiety of withdrawal from heroin, but now I'm doubly afraid of the withdrawal from methadone because I know it's much worse. Several times I have tried a lower dose but I became so nervous and ill that I couldn't sleep and couldn't work and I just had to go back up.

How I would love to wake each morning feeling refreshed and glad to be alive, a natural, healthy, strong young woman. I would love to get married and have children, but I can't plan on these things while I am a slave to this debilitating drug. As I'm over 30 years old I don't have much time, I don't want to let my youth slip away due to my drug dependence.

Sometimes I become fearful that something might happen to me where I won't be able to get my methadone ... I'll get kidnapped or stuck in an elevator for three days and I'll become violently ill and go into convulsions and maybe die. Also I am always afraid that people will find out about my addiction and it will cost me my job or friends.

In other words, I desperately want to detox off of methadone. Until now I've been afraid to try conventional detoxification programs because of the pain and illness which I just can't stand. As you know, I especially have no tolerance to pain, as my body ceased producing endorphins when I became addicted to opiates. Also, with conventional detox methods, patients can take up to two years before they feel normal and can function without cravings, discomfort and anxiety. I just can't afford to drop out of work and life for a long period of illness and recuperation.

EFFECTS OF DRUG MAINTENANCE

Long-acting methadone, LAAM, is now being given in some centres to reduce the numbers of times addicts need to attend, from daily to twice weekly. But Dr Barry Stimmel, Dean of Mount Sinai School of Medicine in New York, reports that:

> Several multicenter studies, sponsored by the National Institute on Drug Abuse, have shown the use of LAAM to be associated with poor patient acceptance and a higher attrition rate than treatment with methadone ... [There is also] disquieting evidence ... concerning the cardiac toxicity of this drug ... Nevertheless, the National Institute on Drug Abuse proceeded to fund Phase II studies, most of which are neither randomised nor controlled, and, presently, is continuing to develop the use of this drug.[296]

Dr David Ausubel of Rockland Children's Psychiatric Center in New York State reported the effects of methadone maintenance treatments in 1983 after an in-depth analysis. He concluded:

(1) that methadone keeps the users in a state of mild euphoria and dulled perceptions, which makes it difficult for them to learn to cope with the inevitable problems of the real world;

(2) that it does not really satisfy the drug-addict's craving for a 'high' so they tend still, whenever possible, to use heroin or other drugs which give a better high;

(3) that it is the addict's personality that craves this high and it is not a real physiological need in the way that diabetics, for example, need insulin in order to enable them to function normally;

(4) that official evaluation studies of methadone maintenance grossly exaggerate its effectiveness;

(5) that methadone maintenance has inadvertently created incomparably more primary methadone addicts than it has cured heroin addicts (see Appendix II, note 1).[22]

In this country, Dr Madden of the Alcohol and Drug Dependence Unit in Chester – amongst others – likewise doubts the usefulness of methadone maintenance.[197]

Professor James Q. Wilson, Professor of Government at Harvard University, adds to this:

> One reason that many addicts join drug-treatment programs is that they become sick of the hassle of getting heroin. *Removing the hassle is tantamount to removing an important reason to seek help.* Finally, a society cannot rely on moral suasion to deter young persons from becoming addicts (the preferred libertarian policy) if we say to them, 'Should you find our arguments about the evils of heroin unpersuasive, we will make the drug freely available to you'. Such an argument ceases to be a moral one, and becomes instead a hypocritical one.[346] (my italics)

The Government Advisory Council reported in July 1984, 'There has been increasing questioning of the practice of prescribing controlled drugs to addicts especially on a long-term maintenance basis.'[259] In fact, Diconal, a drug commonly prescribed by GPs in place of heroin, caused more overdose deaths in 1982 than heroin itself.[137]

But neither government nor the medical profession know what to do with addicts if they are not maintained on drugs, because the existing treatment centres are already unable to cope with those requesting treatment, let alone the tens of thousands who do not ask for help because of the absence of any provision which meets their need.

It is now an accepted medical cliché that 'GPs know very little about drugs and alcoholism', and both general practitioners and hospitals are only too happy to pass the victims over to their psychiatric colleagues. The psychiatrists in turn are hopelessly bemused by and divided over the nature of the addiction problem. They cannot agree as to whether it should be classed as a 'disease' or not, whether it can be treated or not, whether it should be treated by 'supportive' drugs or not, whether it can be 'controlled' or not. Even the DHSS itself wrote in its Report published in December 1984 and sent to all hospital and family doctors: 'Few psychiatrists have any specific training or wide experience in the treatment of drug misuse.'[258]

Then why do so many clinics and doctors continue to prescribe methadone and other abused drugs to their patients? Gerry Stimson, a sociologist, and Dr Edna Oppenheimer of the London Institute of Psychiatry, in their 1982 critical analysis of treatment of heroin addiction in Britain report that 'nearly 40 per cent of patients taken on in any one year will still be patients 10 years later'[297]. Drugs and sterile syringes are supplied free to all registered addicts. Our government is not only paying for drugs for registered addicts, but an earlier survey showed that 95 per cent of these addicts were buying and using illicit drugs along with the legal ones.

Some addicts make a lot of money by selling their 100 per cent heroin supplied by drug dependency units (DDUs) and maintaining themselves on smaller doses or cheaper drugs. Clinics have been known to prescribe as much as 1,140 mg (normal single dose is 5 to 10 mg) for one addict to take every day.[299]

The late Alex Trocchi, author of *Cain's Book*, and himself a registered drug-dependant, saw clearly some of the problems of the official approach:

> If a doctor follows the recommendation of the Brain Report and tries to get his patient to accept a prescription for the smallest amount possible of the drug, an absurd situation arises. From the first interview the user feels forced to resort to cunning, to lying, to cheat, to beg, to fawn, in order to ensure adequate supplies. Doctor and patient are involved in a battle of wits in a destructive pseudo-problem, in which all the energies which should have been brought to bear upon the real problem are wastefully dissipated.[320]

Some DDUs who realize the futility of the system are now concentrating on counselling addicts concerning their problems, rather than on drug maintenance.[127] One DDU commented, 'Observations suggest that while such a prescription alleviates the immediate problem of obtaining drugs it reduces the motivation and energy needed to change the individual's situation and he frequently resumes illegal drug use in addition to his prescription after a period of some months.' Another consultant remarked, 'We have maintained by default. Ten years on we have people maintained, but they are created by me and people like me in other Clinics.'[298]

There is little point in giving therapy while the subject's mind is clouded with drugs. In addition, many who are maintained on methadone feel continually below par from the drug itself, and all of them find it very much harder to discontinue methadone than heroin. This has been noted by expert researchers, one of whom stated categorically: 'The tragedy of methadone is that we cannot get people off methadone.'[212]

> Larry, 42, had been injecting heroin and cocaine intravenously in very large doses for 20 years. He was then transferred by his doctor to methadone (Physeptone) tablets, and for five years before his NET treatment had been given 500 milligrams (100 tablets) of methadone daily and legally by the same doctor. He had been admitted to hospital 15 times in attempts to stop his addiction, without success, and he did not believe it was possible to be cured by electrical stimulation or any other means. After being successfully detoxified by NET he was still off all drugs two years later.

Drug substitution

Every few months, an article appears in a medical journal claiming that some new drug is effective in minimizing withdrawal symptoms of those who attempt to stop their drug-habit. Some drugs such as clonidine and lofexidine do lessen the acute symptoms of the first few days, but all drugs used for this purpose have some unwanted, sometimes dangerous, side-effects.[30, 83] Additionally, no follow-up of patients withdrawn from methadone by means of such drugs has so far been published.

Doctors at Yale University School of Medicine report 'The withdrawal symptoms of anxiety, restlessness, insomnia and muscular aching were most resistant to clonidine treatment and were reported by the majority of patients.'[53] Also, 'Abrupt withdrawal of clonidine is often followed by rebound sympathetic overactivity with symptoms such as anxiety, sweating and tremor, and sometimes severe hypertension. This may occur after only one or two missed doses, and even after gradual withdrawal over 3 days.'[14]

Other experienced researchers in New York have reported, 'Clonidine did not produce euphoria or a positive mood state ... [The] majority ... complained of difficulty in falling asleep. Dry mouth, sluggishness, depression, and occasional bone pain were more infrequent complaints. Systolic and diastolic blood pressure remained significantly decreased throughout the nine days.'[115] However, some British doctors are now finding that clonidine itself has dependency-producing effects.

One of the latest drugs to be recommended as a substitute for opioids is buprenorphine (Temgesic) but already disturbing reports are being received about its potential for physical dependence. A doctor writing to the *British Medical Journal* remarked: 'We have a patient with a history of addiction to alcohol and dipipanone (Diconal) for whom the latter drug was replaced with buprenorphine. The end result of a harrowing story is that he is now firmly addicted to buprenorphine and our attempts to wean him off it have so far been unsuccessful.'[43]

And, just as alcoholics are prescribed Antabuse (disulfiram) to give them a violent physical reaction on drinking alcohol, so some centres now prescribe an oral narcotic antagonist, naltrexone (similar to the injectable naloxone), to be taken regularly after drug-withdrawal, so that acute withdrawal symptoms would occur if the addict weakened and again took an opioid drug. This policy further weakens the addict's already weakened will-power, and so delays his learning to take responsibility for himself and for those whose lives are affected by his actions.

Jimmy Greaves, one of the greats of British football and now a TV personality, speaks feelingly of his experience with aversion drugs, which he had implanted twice to give long-term aversion to alcohol.

> It doesn't stop you thinking alcoholic and that's what you've got to get rid of before you can be cured. You can be off the drink for months and yet, subconsciously, be planning a collision with the stuff somewhere up ahead. The implant, which has a time span attached to its effect, encourages that thinking. I don't believe in it.[209]

Further, according to Dr Cushman, Professor of Pharmacology in Wisconsin, 'Unfortunately, experiences with naltrexone treatment showed that adherence to the full schedule of medications was unusual ... treatment outcomes were far from satisfactory ... These data indicate that routine use of naltrexone in the protocol was not a success in terms of meeting patients' continuing needs. ... Upon stopping naltrexone, many patients relapse.' In addition, 'it has been suggested that long-term use (of naltrexone) may adversely affect function of endogenous opioids.'[81]

This viewpoint is emphasized by Dr Barry Stimmel, Dean at Mount Sinai School of Medicine in New York, pointing out that 'controlled studies assessing this drug (naltrexone) in chronic narcotic dependency have confirmed its relative ineffectiveness, with the proportion of patients remaining in treatment after nine months of therapy not exceeding that of controls'[296].

Substitution of one drug for another is not limited to treating heroin addicts. It is now standard practice by doctors when treating alcoholism to use other drugs - often addictive - such as Heminevrin, Valium or Ativan. Quite apart from the addictive consequences of such drugs, there is also the danger of adverse drug interaction when the effects of one drug are increased or decreased by the previous or simultaneous administration of another drug.

Britain lags behind other countries where there are a number of experimental 'non-medical centres' where the pill-prescribing doctor is no longer the focal point in the cure of the alcohol addict. The Addiction Research Fund (ARF) of Ontario, Canada, has tried several programmes and eventually they set up a centre with no permanent medical staff. After 50,000 admissions and no drug treatment whatsoever, no more than 5 per cent had been referred to hospital and there was not one case of DTs. The Coordinator of ARF said: 'Not only do they recover more quickly, but the majority of withdrawal symptoms don't recur.'

I am aware of the problems of convulsions associated with withdrawal from certain chemicals of abuse. I am simply warning against the present widespread use of addictive drugs by doctors in drug and alcohol treatment centres - which make as many addicts as cure them.

The chronic withdrawal syndrome

But the most important criticism of these drugs in withdrawal is that they seem to have no effect at all on the chronic withdrawal syndrome,[15, 53, 115, 116] which can last as long as one and a half years after stopping methadone.[80]

Two experts from the New York State Substance Abuse Services wrote in 1982:

> After detoxifying, a significant proportion of heroin addicts may experience long-lasting drug craving. Moreover, many complain of decreased feelings of well-being - 'not feeling right' - including feeling empty, uncomfortable, restless, tired and weak, apathetic, hypochondriacal, hypercritical of others, and less efficient ... Craving and its associated malaise - almost a low grade chronic depressive state - are believed to underlie the tendency of many ex-addicts to relapse even after long periods of abstention from use ... there is increasing physiological evidence that significant and persistent changes in the functioning of the body as a result of long-term heroin use are the major factors in relapse behaviour.[191]

The same authors go on to say 'detoxification fails as a treatment procedure for heroin-dependent individuals because it has not been found successful in producing satisfactory retention rates and lasting absence from opiates ... *The term detoxification is a misnomer* ... A more accurate term would be supervised withdrawal' (my italics). In contrast NET is a true detoxification (see Chapter 8).

The chronic withdrawal syndrome (sometimes called the protracted abstinence syndrome) is the term used to describe the long-term dysphoria experienced by everyone who has become dependent on any type of psychoactive drug. It is probably the most important chemical factor in recidivism. It does not make people feel acutely ill – but they say that they just do not feel well. (Details of the effects with various drugs are given in Appendix III.)

Researchers have shown that it takes at least six months to return to physiological normality after stopping heroin,[237] and two to three months for EEG (brain) patterns to return to normal following methadone withdrawal.[274] Symptoms may continue for up to two years after stopping Valium and similar tranquillizers[21]; methadone (Physeptone)[80] and alcohol[321] may take as long as one and a half years. In fact, a physician, alcoholic for only three years, reported recently in the *British Medical Journal* that after stopping drinking completely, 'it was two years before memory fully returned and rational thinking approached normality'[193].

At present, little hope is held out for illicit drug-users unless they are prepared to stay a minimum of one to one and a half years in a long-term therapeutic community – and that after being withdrawn from drugs, usually in a hospital. Staff of Phoenix House in New York, a well-known and large therapeutic community (there is a Phoenix House in Britain also), report that 'over 50 per cent of those who had remained *a year or longer in residence* were successful across five years of follow-up' (my italics), but their criteria of success included methadone maintenance. They go on to say that 'when effectiveness is defined in terms of heroin or methadone abstinence, less than 10 per cent are judged successful, 10 years after treatment'[85].

Such long-term residency, of course, is not cost-effective, and means that only a very small proportion of addicts can be treated, with no provision at all for the many who are hooked on legal tranquillizers or sleeping-pills. Moreover, such a long-term stay tends to make the residents institutionalized and unable to cope on their own with the vagaries of ordinary living when they return to the outside world.

The problem stated

The official Report of the Council of Europe (Strasbourg, 1970) represented by countries studying the drug problems of Europe concluded 'in all countries there has been an upsurge in the number of drug dependants which has now attained the dimensions of an epidemic', and went on to state:

It is important to have in mind that this subject includes not only psychological and medical but also social, educational, cultural and political aspects. The increase in the dimensions of the problem can be looked upon as a symptom that there is something very wrong with society.

The problem is a problem neither of youth nor one of drugs, but a problem of a whole society and an entire life-style shared by young and old alike.

They then made the following recommendations.

In the light of the information received from the national health administrations and of the findings by the members of the team, it appears that the spread of drug dependence has reached epidemic proportions in the 19 countries surveyed.

This epidemic is still increasing and, in view of the lack of complete, accurate and up-to-date information, there is no possibility of forecasting its course, dimensions and duration.

Bearing in mind the importance of drug dependence in Europe and in view of the fact that:

(a) drug dependence is spreading alarmingly and rapidly amongst juveniles (in some European cities at least 25 percent of juvenile groups are at present involved) and that new patterns in drug dependence among juveniles are developing;

(b) drug dependence is increasing in whole populations, especially dependence on those drugs which are not yet under international narcotics control;

(c) there is real danger of the formation of a whole sub-culture;

(d) there is a serious lack of information;

(e) a detailed program is needed if prevention and treatment are to be successful.

While considering that the actual facts of the problem are changing from month to month, the study group feels the necessity for carrying out further studies in the field and for taking immediate measures.

It therefore brings the following recommendations to the attention of the governments concerned.

Information

1 It is recommended that, in each member country, data relating to different types of drug dependence and the personal status of the

drug dependant should be collected on a local, national and European level, on the basis of a European standardized questionnaire. Such a questionnaire should be drawn up under the responsibility of the Council of Europe. A regular exchange of information collected on the basis of such a questionnaire should be organized and maintained on local, national and European levels. In every country an appropriate organ should be set up to collect and evaluate the information and to advise the government in so far as is necessary.

Research

2 With a view to prevention and treatment in each country concerned, experts in the field of drug dependence should be appointed to carry out prospective epidemiological studies and other research projects (i.e. psychic and physical dependence, biochemistry and pharmacological aspects, personality of the drug dependant, group dynamics of adolescent drug users, new methods for education of the public and the professions concerned with this problem).

Treatment

3 Considering the lack of adequate treatment facilities for drug dependants, hospital beds should be made available as urgently as possible. In addition, new special institutions for treatment and after-care should be set up for rehabilitation. Particular attention should be paid to the training of specialized staff able to carry out the treatment.

Prevention

4 In each of the countries concerned, continuous prospective research should be undertaken to detect from the outset new trends in drug abuse, with a view to taking immediate and coordinated preventive measures.

5 Public opinion should be kept currently informed of the dangers of drug dependence. Private agencies should be established with governmental assistance to advise on and prepare material, designed for the information of the population. Well-conceived educational programmes are essential for successful prevention through mass media, schools and clubs, in cooperation with juveniles, parents, teachers, psychologists, social workers, psychiatrists and ex-addicts. Supervised studies should check the efforts and the success of preventive endeavours.

6 Consultative centres should be available for juveniles who are anxious to obtain professional advice on and assistance in their efforts

to free themselves from the danger of a tendency toward drug dependence, without fear of penal prosecution.

7 While the drug-abuser - whether a beginner or already dependent - is a medical problem, the drug trafficker is a legal one and severe punitive measures should be taken against anyone who derives profit from the craving of the dependent individual or seduces the uninitiated to become drug dependent.

Coordination

8 An appropriate centre in one of the member States of the Council of Europe should be entrusted with:

(a) the collection and dissemination of information;

(b) the coordination of national research at an international level and promotion of joint research;

(c) new proposals for research, prevention and treatment programmes.

To the best of my knowledge, no serious attempt - if any - has been made by the 19 countries who produced these recommendations, or others, to implement, investigate or propose a comparable solution to a social evil 'of epidemic proportions' - even though it often involves the families of the very legislators, statesmen and politicians who draw up the programmes, or even themselves.

Chapter 3
Lay introduction to NET

Stress

Stress affects all kinds and classes of people, from highly paid executives and rock musicians to housekeepers and teenagers.

The symptoms of stress are well known: anxiety, headaches, sleeplessness, irritation, sweaty palms, urge to urinate, memory blanks, mental and physical pain.

Our bodies are so constructed that every form of stress alerts the brain to produce a substance to deal with that impulse. For example, in war, or sport, or business, or during a family quarrel, when we feel anxiety, or stress, or fear, our brains - which were quietly ticking over at 8 to 12 cycles per second before the stress impulse - suddenly switch to a high frequency of 13 to 21 cycles per second. This triggers certain cells to produce natural chemical substances which help us to meet and overcome the problem, such as the hormone adrenaline for 'fight or flight', or the recently discovered endorphins - produced by the brain - for circumstances involving pain or emotion.

Our brain cells have the capacity to produce all sorts of chemicals when required. But if, instead of meeting or resolving a problem, we panic or are defeated by it and run to the doctor (or cigarette vending-machine, or off-licence, or drug dealer, or pharmacist) for some form of synthetic chemical, and we introduce this to the body, the brain immediately gets the message that the natural substance need no longer be produced. Often the effects of the chemical are more serious than the stress condition itself. Then, when we try to stop taking the medicine, or cigarette, or drug, or alcohol, we suffer a 'drug hunger', 'withdrawal' or 'craving'. We are on our way to addiction.

NeuroElectric Therapy

Over the years since 1973 I have developed a technique which has been remarkably successful in helping many people overcome a wide range of addictions. It is called NET, which stands for NeuroElectric Therapy.

NET itself is not a cure for addiction, but it is an effective detoxification of addictions of all kinds - the first to be discovered. For centuries alcoholics, drug addicts and drug dependants wishing to drop their habit have had to 'dry out' or go 'cold turkey', or even take another, more addictive, drug as a supposed cure. Now, for the first time it is possible for addicts to be detoxified from any chemical form of addiction, in only 10 days, with minimal discomfort. NET is also the first treatment ever to reverse the long-term chronic withdrawal syndrome, which may last for many months, in addition to dealing with the acute withdrawal syndrome.

This detoxification is accomplished by a pocket-size transistorized machine. The machine, with its quadrillion possible combinations of frequencies and wave-forms, launches a new scientific system of medicine which no longer drugs the body with chemicals in treatment, but stimulates body cells to produce their own natural chemical substances.

The small portable stimulator, similar in appearance to a 'Walkman' cassette tape-player often worn by joggers, has two leads which attach to adhesive electrodes fitted behind the ears. These carry a current, which gives a slight, not unpleasant, tingling sensation, and the patient uses it almost continuously for the 10 days of treatment.

RATIONALE OF NET

So how does NET work?

Some people may have heard or read of the endorphins, the brain's natural pain-killers. For instance, if you are a jogger, your endorphin production increases dramatically while you are running and makes you feel elated. Production of endorphins also increases in response to pain. But when the body becomes accustomed to taking a drug, for example heroin, the endorphins stop being formed because the sites (receptors) on the brain cells where endorphins normally attach to produce their effects are always full of heroin. These sites have to be empty before the brain starts producing endorphins again.

We now know that the correct kind of electrical current will send a message to the brain to produce these endorphins again, and from my experience, over 12 years, it takes 10 days of stimulation with most people for the brain to take over this function normally. That is why an average of 10 days NET is required, although a few people need less time and a few need longer.

A description of the procedure involved at our first clinic will illustrate the application of NET in treatment.

CLINIC FOR NET

The manor house in which our first clinic was set up could accommodate 25 patients in shared or single rooms and had a large lounge, dining room and recreation room for common use. Various indoor games were available and tennis, croquet, swimming and fishing were possible in the grounds. Most patients stayed from 15 to 40 days, with the emphasis in the first 10 days being on detoxification, followed by a month of counselling to help the detoxified individuals find new meaning in life. It was hoped that such counselling would enable them to re-enter ordinary society with the capacity to function adequately without drugs.

The clinic was designed to treat all types of chemical or behavioural tendencies and addictions, associated neural conditions and chronic pain. Residents could be accepted while on probation, direct from prison, or while on trial if circumstances warranted. For inpatient treatment we could accept employed people only if they could obtain at least 10 days' leave for the first phase. We were prepared to consider couples, under special circumstances, or minors, with parental consent. We did not accept psychotic or schizophrenic patients, and could not at that time accept patients with severe physical disabilities. Patients who left without permission were not readmitted without a multidisciplinary discussion of the reasons for their departure. As we said in our official descriptive literature about the clinic, however, 'No patient will be left without hope of treatment.'

Admission procedures could be initiated by the individual, his or her doctor, a friend or member of the family, or any addiction organization by telephone or letter. Reports on the individual's history or condition were considered useful but not essential at the time of initial assessment by the senior medical consultant. Applicants were given leaflets or pamphlets describing the clinic, ground rules, and both the nature and philosophy of our treatment.

Referral agencies or immediate relatives were invited to visit the clinic to see it for themselves before the selection interview. Although the patient's motivation was not an essential factor for acceptance, it did influence our decision about an admission date. This first clinic was so successful, despite teething problems, that although it had to close in 1981 through lack of financial support, all future clinics will follow a similar pattern.

Before admission we have a long interview with the patient and spouse or close relatives. Addicts are assured that all they say to the doctor or counsellor will remain confidential but they should be encouraged to tell the full story of their addiction to their spouse or parents, because learning to speak the whole truth is part of the healing process. I begin the first interview by saying that 'All drug-addicts and alcoholics become habitual liars because of the necessity to cover up their actions. So I shall weigh up everything you tell me in the light of my own experience and then decide for myself if I think it is true or not.' This approach usually produces an immediate reaction of relief, because the constant deceits and subterfuges are a problem to them, whether admitted or not.

After all medical, personal and family details are ascertained, the treatment is briefly described. When patients arrive for admission they are asked to hand over all drugs. No drugs at all are given during NET treatment unless some medical condition requires them. Even sleeping-pills and tranquillizers are forbidden because every such pill-taking is followed by a period of rebound insomnia or anxiety, and thus only prolongs discomfort. Further, the body has become so tolerant to drugs that the amount needed to ensure sleep would be dangerously near an overdose.

The hardest part is the first few nights of poor sleep. Again, a few patients have slept well from the start, but most do not develop a normal sleep pattern until between the third and ninth nights. Without NET, it takes about two months to achieve normal sleep after stopping heroin or alcohol, and up to four months after barbiturates.

TECHNIQUE

Adhesive electrodes are attached behind the ears, and wires connect to the stimulator, which hooks on to a belt or is put in a pocket. It is worn all the time, day and night - even while playing tennis

- but, of course, taken off while swimming or showering. From the seventh day we start weaning patients off the stimulator, according to response to treatment. Most feel physically normal, healthy and energetic at some point before the 10 days are finished, but a few say it has taken one to three weeks after finishing NET before they feel completely healthy.

Patients walk around from the first day and are expected to take part in all activities, including household duties, as part of the therapy. Outdoor work, such as gardening, helps most. Nurses are available in the night to talk to those having trouble with sleeplessness.

About the fourth or fifth day, patients often become euphoric because they have succeeded in getting off drugs and are feeling well without them, but this is followed by a sudden recognition of the emptiness of life without drugs - like losing a husband or wife. At this point help from an understanding counsellor is provided, mostly on an individual basis but also in groups. Then begins a further 30-day period of rehabilitation specifically planned for each patient's needs. At this stage family and/or spouse are always requested to participate in counselling for themselves as well as for the patient.

Only a few of my patients have claimed that they have had no withdrawal symptoms at all - and these have all been very heavy users. Most say that NET keeps symptoms 'at bay', with only the feeling of the onset of a common cold. Discomfort remains bearable and everything possible is done to ease it. Hard exercise, hot baths and massage reduce the discomfort considerably.

The clinical evidence is that NET not only ameliorates the acute symptoms of withdrawal but also abolishes the chronic withdrawal syndrome within one to three weeks instead of the usual many months, even years.

The science behind NET is complicated. Readers interested in understanding more about the technique should turn to Part II, which explains in detail how I developed the stimulator.

For those less scientifically inclined, the following section should be sufficient.

Independent summary of NET clinical research

In 1982, *Omni*, an American-based science magazine, had heard of my work and after a 10-month investigation, in which the

Omni associate editor Kathleen McAuliffe indefatigably and meticulously interrogated patients, colleagues, interested and sceptical doctors and scientists, they published a major article in the January 1983 issue. Because it gives an independent and admirable survey of NET based on exhaustive investigation, I have asked Kathleen McAuliffe and the editors of *Omni* magazine for permission to reprint an edited version of the article.

> 'It looks like a Walkman,' explains Pete Townshend, the lead guitarist and chief songwriter for The Who, the British rock band. 'You clip this transistor-size unit onto your belt, and there's two wires leading from it that you attach behind your ears. Then it's a question of tuning in to the right frequency.'
>
> The 38-year-old rock star is not describing the latest advance in recording technology, but a novel treatment for drug addiction – a treatment that may work by striking a melodic chord in the brain. The Walkman look-alike transmits a tiny electrical signal that appears to harmonize with natural brain rhythms and, in the process, reduce craving and anxiety. Or at least it worked for Townshend. The little black box, he says, saved him from a nearly suicidal two-year alcoholic binge that eventually drove him to heavy tranquillizers and virtually any other drug he could lay his hands on. 'The treatment works not only for boozers,' Townshend emphasizes. 'It's helped people give up cigarettes, heroin, barbiturates, speed, cocaine, marijuana – you name it. There is a different frequency that works best for each kind of addiction.'
>
> Dr Margaret Patterson, a Scottish surgeon, is the owner and inventor of this magical device. Her black box sounds suspiciously like quackery. Just twiddle a few knobs and – presto – you can be cured of every imaginable vice. But the magic is real to people in the Rock 'n' Roll industry, who call her a miracle worker. Apparently Townshend is not the only celebrity who has benefited from her unusual remedy. She is credited with having reformed more than a dozen top recording stars, including ex-heroin addicts Eric Clapton and the seemingly indestructable Keith Richards, of the Rolling Stones, whose reckless abuse of drugs became as legendary as his music.
>
> Happily, Dr Patterson does not fit the image of either a charlatan or a cult figure. She is in her 50s, slender of frame, with a kindly face that radiates compassion. Her pale blue eyes are set off by a magnificent mane of auburn hair, which is swept up into a graceful, oversized bun. 'I hesitate to use the word "*cure*",' she says in a soft, lilting burr. 'I prefer to call it a method of rapid detoxification. The electricity quickly cleanses the addict's system of drugs, restoring the

body to normal within ten days. Most patients report that their craving also subsides in the process.'

Over the last decade in Britain, almost 300 addicts have received NeuroElectric Therapy (NET), the technical name for her treatment. Dr Patterson claims that all but four were left drug-free at the end of the detoxification process - a remarkable 98 per cent success rate. 'NET should not be confused with ECT (electroconvulsive therapy) for mentally ill patients,' she cautions. 'NET is far milder, involving currents at least twenty times weaker. Patients feel only a slight tingling sensation behind their ears where the electrodes are taped on.' Yet this 'mild' therapy, she insists, will subdue the violent physiological reactions that can make 'going cold turkey' intolerable for even the most strong-willed person. Though normally soft-spoken, Patterson asserts unequivocally, 'I can take anyone off a drug of abuse, no matter how severe his or her addiction, with only minimal discomfort.'

Of course, not all those who complete the detoxification program remain abstinent. Patterson emphasizes that NET is most effective when backed up by counselling, remedial training, and supportive home environment. For many individuals, however, the treatment does appear to have long-lasting effects. If we are to believe the recidivism figures she cites, they are many times lower than the national average for every class of addictive drug.

A glance at Patterson's credentials provides reassurance that she is both serious and highly capable. At 21, she was the youngest woman to qualify as a doctor at Scotland's Aberdeen University. Only four years later she obtained her fellowship at the Royal College of Surgeons at Edinburgh University - an elite circle that few penetrate before their 30s. And just before her 40th birthday she was presented one of her native land's highest honors by the Queen - an M.B.E., or Member of the British Empire - for her outstanding medical work in India.

Colleagues and patients describe the tiny Scottish surgeon as warm, confident, and virtually unflappable. 'You can't con her,' says one patient who has spent years cheating and lying to get bigger drug prescriptions. 'And if you try to put one over on her, she won't turn her back on you like other doctors.'

'She's the sort of mother you always dreamed of having,' says a female addict. Still another views her as a saintly figure 'with the selfless devotion of someone like Mother Theresa.'

Patterson's close rapport with her patients has made some professionals question whether her dazzling record in drug rehabilitation is really attributable to the powers of electricity. 'It's her personality' is the chief disclaimer psychiatrists have attached to her work. 'She doesn't control for psychological factors such as people's expectations,' says Dr Richard B. Resnick, an associate professor at New York Medical College, who is recognized as an innovator in the treatment of heroin addiction. 'For example, what happens if you fasten electrodes to patients' heads but don't turn on the electricity? You just talk to them and feed them chicken soup. Will they do better, the same, or worse than the group that got current?'

Such skepticism is less common in England, where Dr Patterson's clinical practice was based until recently. There, a number of doctors have already begun to obtain the same beneficial effects with her electrical stimulator model.

Dr Margaret Cameron, a psychiatrist in Somerset, England, reports that NET gives 'very, very good results - better than any other treatment I've encountered.' Since May 1981, Dr Cameron has treated 40 alcoholics, two methadone addicts, four heroin addicts, and a few individuals with mixed addictions involving cocaine and barbiturates. In follow-up interviews conducted six months to a year later, 60 per cent of the alcoholics were still off alcoholic beverages and none of the other patients had relapsed. A private practitioner based in New Jersey, Dr Joseph Winston, shares Cameron's enthusiasm for NET. 'As a benign, effective technique for withdrawing people from drugs, it is virtually unmatched.'

If NET has met with resistance, it is because its mode of action strains the explanatory powers of modern science. Until recently, orthodox medicine refused to recognize that infinitesimal electrical currents may influence the behavior or function of living organisms. Currents less than 100 millivolts - or below the threshold for triggering a nerve impulse - were assumed to have no effect on biological processes. This dogmatic view had to be reassessed when accounts of such unsettling phenomena began appearing with increasing frequency in technical journals over the last decade. NET is, in fact, only one branch of a young, controversial discipline that is still struggling to achieve respectability, the science of electrical medicine.

In the early 1970s scientists began introducing very small currents via electrodes to different parts of the body - with dramatic results. A rat amputee was induced to regrow a forelimb down to midjoint, according to one exciting - though sometimes contested - report. In human applications, the FDA has approved the use of such currents for stitching together bone fractures. Recent experimental trials also indicate that trickling flows of electricity promote the healing of chronic bed-sores, burns, and even peripheral-nerve injuries. The external currents, it is theorized, stimulate rapid healing by augmenting the body's internal currents.

'By contrast, weak currents applied to the brain affect different physiological processes,' says Dr Robert O. Becker, a pioneer of electrical medicine who recently retired from Veterans Administration Hospital, in Syracuse, New York. 'But I believe Dr Patterson is producing profound alterations of the central nervous system. The psychological set that makes a person become an addict seems to disappear.'

Researchers are now starting to elucidate NET's scientific rationale, winning over new converts from the more conservative ranks of the medical profession. In the process, Dr Patterson's black box is helping to unlock the mysterious inner workings of that other black box: the human brain. The stimulus goes in and the response comes out, but seldom are we afforded a glimpse of what happens in between. By probing NET's effects on experimental animals, investigators are shedding light on the underlying mechanisms that control everything from addictive behaviors to our most basic drives and emotions. As Dr Becker surmised, the stimulator does indeed cause 'profound alterations of the nervous system.' Underlying consciousness is an intricate orchestral arrangement of trillions of brain cells, firing in concert. Like different instruments in a symphony, subpopulations of neurones are now believed to produce frequencies within a specific range. Frequency, so to speak, is the music of the hemispheres.

Like penicillin and X-rays, NET was born of scientific serendipity. It began with an accidental discovery in the autumn of 1972. At that time Dr Patterson was head of surgery at Hong Kong's Tung Wah Hospital, a large charity institution with poor clientele. A neurosurgeon colleague, Dr H. L. Wen, had just returned from the People's Republic of China, where he had learned the techniques of electro-acupuncture. Primarily interested in its usefulness in the suppression of pain, he began testing it on patients with a variety of ills. Dr Wen, however, did not know that almost 15 percent of his patients were addicted to heroin or opium of extremely high purity. At that time their drugs were easily affordable at a daily cost of less than a pack of cigarettes.

'One day', Patterson recalls, 'an addict approached Dr Wen, announcing that the electro-acupuncture had stopped his withdrawal symptoms. "I felt as if I'd just had a shot of heroin," he said. Wen initially thought nothing of it, but a few hours later another addict reported a similar experience, equating the electro-acupuncture with a certain dosage of opium.'

Further inquiries revealed that a few alcoholics and cigarette smokers in Wen's experimental group had also been freed from their craving. To the eye, however, the electro-acupuncture produced the most dramatic response in the narcotics addicts deprived of their drugs. The characteristic runny nose, stomach cramps, aching joints, and feeling of anxiety usually disappeared after 10 to 15 minutes stimulation by needles inserted inside the hollow of the external ear, at the acupuncturist's lung point. At first these good effects lasted only a few hours. But with repeated treatments, patients remained symptom-free for periods of longer duration.

The results of Wen's first study with 40 opiate addicts were published in the *Asian Journal of Medicine* the following spring. Of this group, 39 were drug-free by the time they left the hospital, roughly two weeks after starting treatment. When Dr Patterson returned to England in July 1973, however, she found that addicts were far less enthusiastic about the procedure. The Chinese loved acupuncture; the British hated it. 'As bizarre as it may sound,' Patterson explains, 'Westerners - even those who mainlined drugs - often had an aversion to needles.'

There was another reason not to use the needles. Patterson had suspected from the outset that acupuncture was essentially an electrical phenomenon. Even the traditional explanation hinted that this might be so. The ancient practice revolves around the notion that all living things possess vital energy, called *chi*, which circulates through the body by way of a network of channels, or 'meridians.' Sickness was seen to be the result of disharmony, manifested by an obstruction in the flow of *chi*, which the needling was thought to remedy.

Was *chi* the ancients' concept for what modern man now recognizes as the internal currents that course through the body? Could it be that the Chinese, more than 2,500 years before the discovery of electricity, had intuitively sought to alter this life force in an attempt to alleviate pain and to cure disease? Perhaps, Dr Patterson reasoned, the twirling of needles generates a tiny electrical voltage. Viewed in this light, the more recent practice of electro-acupuncture was simply a more intense form of the original twirling technique. If so, the electrical signal would be of crucial significance in the treatment of addictions.

Years of clinical trial and error eventually confirmed her hunch. First Dr Patterson replaced the needles with electrodes. Then she went on to compare direct current with alternating current, while varying the voltage, shape, and other aspects of the electrical signal. Next she altered the electrode placement, finding a position just behind the ear over the mastoid bone to be more effective than the lung point. But, of all the variables explored, electrical frequency quickly emerged as the single most important element for success. Those addicted to narcotics and sedatives preferred frequencies within the 75 Hz to 300 Hz range, barbiturate addicts responded to lower frequencies, and still other addicts, especially those dependent on cocaine and amphetamines, benefited most from frequencies as high as 2000 Hz. 'Musicians,' she fondly recalls, 'really helped to strengthen my guesswork during those early days. They invariably found the correct therapeutic setting right away. It was as if their brains were more attuned to frequency.'

A further refinement of the therapy was prompted by still another fortuitous discovery: A heavy abuser fell asleep with the stimulator on and awoke 30 hours later, well-rested and eager to take Dr Patterson's children ice-skating. From that moment onward, she advocated continuous current application in the initial phases of treatment. She began the search for more comfortable electrodes that could be worn during sleep and for smaller electrical simulators that could be clipped onto belts, permitting mobility during the day.

By 1976, Dr Patterson had transformed electro-acupuncture into an exciting new experimental treatment mode that she christened NeuroElectric Therapy. In her first clinical study, which was reported that year in the U.N. *Bulletin on Narcotics*, opiate addicts given NET as in-patients were all found to be drug-free an average of 10 months after completing treatment. In contrast, opiate addicts who received NET only during the day as out-patients did not fare as well: 47 percent were drug-free at the time of the follow-up.

Because this preliminary investigation was limited to 23 patients, her results could not be extrapolated to a larger cross section of addicts. To provide better information about the long-term effects of NET, and also to assess its value in the treatment of other kinds of addictions, Dr Patterson was recently awarded a research grant by the British Medical Association.

In the autumn of 1982, at a Washington, D.C. symposium sponsored by the American Holistic Medical Association, Dr Patterson presented the findings from this follow-up evaluation, which tracked the progress of patients treated between 1973 and 1980. Data was obtained from confidential questionnaires and, when possible, from personal interviews. Fifty percent responded to the survey, and these respondents included 66 drug addicts (mostly mainline heroin or methadone users and mixed-addiction cases), 9 cigarette smokers, and 18 alcoholics. At the time of the follow-up, total abstinence was said to be achieved by 80 per cent of the alcoholics who stated abstinence to be their goal. An additional seven alcoholics whose goal on admission was 'controlled drinking' all reported success. (As Dr Patterson herself cautions, however, these figures probably represent too favourable an outcome since patients who relapsed, especially alcoholics, may have been less likely to reply to the survey.) Of those who were successfully weaned from their dependence,

68 percent said they never or only rarely experienced craving, 15 percent said they occasionally felt craving, and another 17 percent said they frequently felt craving.

Interestingly, none of the drug addicts at the time of reporting had substituted alcohol for their earlier addiction - a finding that contrasts sharply with the figures cited in other studies. In one national survey, for example, 60 percent of addicts who had given up narcotics became heavy drinkers or alcoholics. Equally noteworthy was the equally low dropout rate of all addicts enrolled in the program: only 1.6 percent did not complete the detoxification.

All things considered, the success of Dr Patterson's patients is probably the most remarkable from the standpoint of the brief duration of the therapy, which, including counseling, rarely extends beyond 30 days. According to a large study of drug abusers admitted to a variety of government sponsored programs, addicts treated less than three months did not fare any better than those in a no-treatment comparison group. So NET seems to achieve in a few weeks what few, if any, orthodox treatments can accomplish after months or years.

Not everyone, however, is convinced by the report's conclusions. A look at the history of drug reform in the United States shows that their cynicism is not ill-founded. Consider the government's efforts to curb narcotics use. The first U.S. Public Health Service hospital for heroin addicts opened in Lexington, Kentucky, where 18,000 patients were admitted between 1935 and 1952. All except some 7 percent of the alumni promptly relapsed after dismissal from the institution - a dreary record that other institutions scarcely improved upon in subsequent decades.

By the 1960s heroin addiction had spread like cancer through inner-city ghettos. To control the expanding epidemic, health professionals turned to methadone, a synthetic opiate that is legally prescribed. Today thousands of clinics throughout the nation dispense methadone to certified addicts, and those maintained in these programs show higher rates of employment and fewer criminal offenses than before they began treatment. But methadone, alas, is even more addictive than heroin. As one medical authority points out, 'The tragedy of methadone is that we cannot get people off methadone.'

For narcotics addicts who aspire to a drug-free existence, society offers two main alternatives: the highly structured and insulated environments of such residential homes as Daytop Village, Phoenix House and Odyssey House or out-patient clinics, which provide daily counseling services. As many as 30 to 40 percent of the people who enroll in these community-based programs remain abstinent a year after leaving treatment. But to enter most of these programs one must first detoxify in a hospital. And here's the hitch: 64 percent don't make it past the acute withdrawal phase to qualify for further treatment.

'It is still not understood why simple detoxification is so ineffective, but the facts are clear and inescapable,' says Dr Avram Goldstein, professor of pharmacology at Stanford University. 'As I see it, the reason for the dismal failure ... is that the newly detoxified addict, still driven by discomfort, physiologic imbalance, and intense craving, cannot focus attention on the necessary first steps toward rehabilitation, but soon succumbs and starts using heroin.'

Jean Cocteau, the French writer, who resumed smoking after medicine had 'purged' him of the habit, put it another way: 'Now that I am cured, I feel empty, poor, heartbroken and ill.'

In sharp contrast, NET patients are said to emerge from treatment feeling healthy, energetic, even cheerful. Dr Joseph Winston, the American physician who collaborated with Dr Patterson in the treatment of Keith Richards, recalls that the musician 'came to us terribly ill. He was literally green. But he slept eighteen hours the first day, and ten days later he was playing tennis, and the group said he had not looked so good in years.'

Surprisingly, many patients who go on to build drug-free lives do not receive any formal counseling beyond that provided during the brief detoxification program. Yet NET, by itself, cannot remove the root causes of addiction, nor can it replace years of maladaption with healthy skills for coping with life's stresses and disappointments. Why then do so many patients experience such a metamorphosis?

The treatment, Dr Patterson believes, simply sets the stage for further growth. 'Because they feel so good,' she says, 'they are better able to face the sort of problems that drove them to addiction in the first place. You see, most people who come off drugs without NET enter a phase of prolonged dysphoria. They suffer from fearful depression and pessimism. They can't eat. They can't sleep. They have no energy. This can last for six months in the case of heroin, and even longer in the case of methadone and barbiturate addiction. But NET restores physiological normality within ten days, which enormously reduces the amount of time needed for readjustment.'

If anything, Dr Patterson thinks that euphoria - not dysphoria - is to blame when rehabilitation fails. The newly detoxified addict is optimistic to the point of being overconfident. 'In their elated state,' Dr Patterson says, 'they think it will be easy to stay off drugs and then end up stumbling, because they don't make enough of an effort to change their ways.'

As if obeying Newtonian mechanics, the black box appears to

counter one mood shift with an equal swing in the opposite direction, until the emotional pendulum finally comes to rest. Is the black box, in reality, an electronic substitute for a chemical high? How can a physical treatment cause such a swing towards euphoria?

As fate would have it, a scientist who had taught Dr Patterson years earlier, Professor Hans Kosterlitz, would once again serve as her mentor by illuminating the mainspring of euphoria in the brain. While working with Dr John Hughes at the University of Aberdeen in 1975, Dr Kosterlitz identified an endorphin, a natural brain chemical, with a molecular structure very similar to the opiates. For this outstanding discovery, the investigators later received the prestigious Lasker Award, revered as America's equivalent of the Nobel Prize in medicine. Almost overnight their finding triggered an explosion in the understanding of the biochemical basis of behavior, opening a new vista on the controlling factors behind addiction. Opium, heroin, morphine, and other related drugs owe their potency to what Avram Goldstein calls 'one of nature's most bizarre coincidences' – their uncanny resemblance to the endorphins.

Over the succeeding years researchers uncovered evidence of myriad other brain hormones that mimic psychoactive drugs, from Valium and angel dust to hallucinogens. Almost every mind-altering substance, it is now assumed, has an analogue in the brain. And the precise mixture of neurojuices in this biochemical cocktail can mean the difference between tripping, speeding, crashing or seeing the world through sober eyes.

These insights immediately suggested how the addict becomes trapped in a nightmarish cycle of dependency. In the initial phases of narcotic use, for example, the individual is assumed to have normal levels of endorphins in the brain. Injecting heroin causes a sudden and drastic elevation of opiates, which is subjectively interpreted as ecstasy. If through repeated use the brain is regularly flooded with opiates, it redresses the imbalance by cutting back on the production of its internal supply. Hence, the well known condition of tolerance develops. The addict steps up his dosage, and the brain further compensates by calling a massive shutdown of production. Eventually, according to the theory, the addict is shooting up solely for the purpose of 'feeling normal'. Should the drug supply be cut off at this stage, the opiate shortage cannot be instantly remedied. Drought ensues, unleashing withdrawal symptoms.

If an exogenous drug depletes the brain of its natural counterpart, it seemed logical that NET might quite literally juice up the system, rapidly replenishing the scarce neurochemical. Might certain frequencies of current catalyze the release of different brain hormones? Dr Patterson wondered.

To find out, she conducted animal experiments in collaboration with biochemist Dr Ifor Capel at the Marie Curie Memorial Foundation Research Department, in Surrey, England. Simply by monitoring the blood of NET-treated rats, the investigators discovered low frequency currents can indeed cause as much as a three-fold elevation of endorphin levels.

In another experiment the researchers examined NET's effects on rats rendered unconscious by massive doses of barbiturates. Once asleep, all the animals had electrodes clipped on to their ears, but only half the group actually received electrical current. The result: At one particular frequency - 10 Hz - the experimental group rapidly regained consciousness, sleeping on average 40 percent less than the rats that received no electricity.

Why is the detoxification process hastened? One clue surfaced when the rats' brain tissue was analyzed. It was learned that the 10 Hz signal speeds up the production and turnover rate of serotonin (a neurotransmitter that acts as a stimulant to the central nervous system).

Similar experiments have now been repeated on rats made unconscious by injecting them with alcohol or ketamine (a cousin of angel dust). In almost every instance the frequencies that reduced sleeping time had earlier been proved therapeutic in the detoxification of human addicts. 'Virtually every single parameter of current that I had stumbled upon during my clinical work was corroborated by the rat studies,' Dr Patterson declares, with barely concealed excitement.

How a weak electrical current can open the floodgates of the mind is still a matter of conjecture, but the implications are obvious. Like a citizen's band transmitter that infiltrates television frequencies, the black box must broadcast through brain frequency channels. And just as a TV receiver can pick up CB transmissions from a passing truck, the brain undoubtedly responds to the foreign-generated signal as if it originated from within its own communication network.

'As far as we can tell,' says Dr Capel, a rugged Welshman with a melodic voice, 'each brain center generates impulses at a specific frequency based on the predominant neurotransmitters it secretes. In other words, the brain's internal communications system - its language - if you like - is based on frequency.'

Unfortunately, neuroscientists are not yet fluent in this new tongue. 'NET is still a very blunt tool,' Capel acknowledges. 'Presumably, when we send in waves of energy at, say 10 Hz, certain cells in the lower brain stem will respond, because they normally fire at that frequency range. As a result, particular mood-altering chemicals associated with that region will be released. That's what we *hope* is happening. In reality, however, much of the signal may be lost before it actually reaches the target cells. We just don't know. But if we can fine-tune the signal I am confident our results will steadily improve.'

Dr Patterson has now begun testing a new, improved model of the stimulator.

Will NET open a new route to salvation for the millions who each year flock to Alcoholics Anonymous, Smoke Enders, and methadone maintenance clinics? Clearly the final verdict is contingent upon replication of controlled studies. But if a feeble electrical current can truly curb the mind's excesses - from uncontrollable lusts to extremes of mood - its impact is due to be far-reaching.

'Addicts may represent only a tiny fraction of the people who will eventually be helped by NET,' Capel predicts. 'In all likelihood it will find an enormous range of uses, especially in the area of pain control.' In one preliminary trial, terminal patients suffering from chronic pain found NET just as effective as their daily dose of morphine. 'By stimulating the brain's own pain-killer, we didn't have to administer drugs,' Capel marvels.

Early data also indicates that NET may prove highly promising in the treatment of mental disorders. The frequencies that induce euphoria and reduce tension, according to Dr Cameron, 'seem to work wonders for patients suffering from severe depression and acute anxiety.' Though it is far too soon to draw any conclusions, she notes that a 'few of the half-dozen chronic depressives we've treated have found themselves jobs after years of unemployment.'

As for Dr Patterson, she hopes eventually to broaden her practice to include behavioral addicts, from overeating and compulsive gambling to video game fanaticism. Absurdity aside, these applications follow a certain logic. 'Her ideas make perfect sense if one accepts the idea that behavioral addictions have a chemical basis,' says Dr William Regelson, at the Medical College of Virginia. 'It is very likely, for example, that all activities vital to survival - from sex to physical exercise - are physiologically addictive. It is now thought that the phenomenon called jogger's high is actually endorphin-mediated. In all probability, eating also releases some kind of pleasurable molecule. After all, why do we crave food? Low blood-sugar levels don't explain why. The truth is that we feel abnormal when we haven't eaten in a while. Some chemical in our brain has become depleted. We become restless and agitated, and, after extreme deprivation, we suffer withdrawal symptoms commonly known as hunger pangs. The only way to relieve our discomfort is to get more food. It's a fix - plain and simple.'

If basic drives are addictive, then drugs are an ingenious means of short-cutting the elaborate scheme nature devised to ensure that we maintain health and reproduce ourselves. Merely by popping a pill, we can top off our neurochemical reservoirs with no sweat expended. Instant orgasm without foreplay. A cheap thrill.

But can't the same be said of NET? 'Is it not, after all, an electronic fix?' asks Regelson, who fears the black box may become addictive in its own right. Dr Patterson has kept her eyes open to any signs that her patients are becoming physically dependent on the equipment. But she rules out the possibility that there will ever be a black market in the black boxes, because individual models can cost upward of $1,000 - hefty sum to cough up for purely recreational use. Besides, she has not encountered a single instance of electronic addiction in her ten years of practice. The explanation, she believes, 'is that drugs - for the very reason that they are foreign - upset the brain's chemistry. NET, on the other hand, simply coaxes the brain to restore its own chemical balance. The body heals itself.'

The intuitive feelings of her patients support this view. As reformed heroin addict Stuart Harris says, 'At first I thought it would be fun to wire up the human race, so we could all go whizzing about. But after the initial buzz, you feel, well, normal. Frankly, all NET does is to help you face reality.'

Dr Patterson concurs: 'All we can do is give people a chance. We can get them off whatever drug they're hooked to, but it's up to them to fill the void. They've got to find a constructive substitute for the drugs that have dominated their lives.'[226]

Placebos

As this extract shows, throughout the development of NET I have had my fair share of detractors. The strongest lobby has come from psychiatrists who try to explain the success of NET in the terms of the 'placebo effect'.

While it is known what a placebo is, how a placebo works is not fully understood. A placebo is an inert substance used to test new drugs in medical trials. However, it is coming to be realized that placebos not only can be made to appear like medicines but can also act like medicine in a way that baffles scientists. Placebos have even been known to 'cure' malignant conditions and it is for this reason that doctors and scientists are highly suspicious of medicines like Laetrile, which has been claimed, without proof, to be a cancer cure.

The 'placebo effect' was the reason most often given by some psychiatrists and doctors to explain away my apparent successes. None of them, incidentally, had ever been in touch with me; or, from the impression gathered from their comments in the media when they were interviewed regarding my work, had they even read about it.

Another medical consensus about my work with NET even went so far as to maintain that my successes could be explained by the fact that I was 'a healer'. I can well imagine the kind of response I would have had from the same group of doctors had I made personal claims to being 'a healer'!

The witty and penetrating writer Adam Smith, in his book, *Powers of Mind,* said:

> Placebo is *I shall be pleasing* in Latin, and nothing at all in pharmacology. It is a fake. Sugar and water. It's there to fool the mind. Of course, you have to believe the placebo is real, and clever psychologists have even tested what is most real in their nothing pill ... The clever psychologists compared placebos and pain relievers in a double blind test, where neither the experimenter nor pill taster knew what was what, and the placebo were 50-something per cent as effective as practically everything! 54 per cent as aspirin, 54 per cent as Darvon (a tranquillizer (sic)), 56 per cent as morphine. Two placebos work better than one. Placebo injections work better than placebo pills. Placebos work better when they aren't given by doctors because doctors like to give real medicine and not sugar pills, and the patient gets the unverbalized message from the doctor's face and tone: the vibes give it away.[289]

The word 'placebo' has been used since 1811 to describe an inert, innocuous medication, or 'medicine given more to please than to benefit the patient'. In other words, a 'dummy tablet'. The term is also used of a doctor with 'an effective bedside manner', a warm personality, an enthusiastic conviction.

NORMAN COUSINS' EXPERIENCE

The placebo effect was also claimed by reactionary doctors to explain the remarkable recovery of Norman Cousins, the distinguished editor of *Saturday Review.* Flying home to the United States from a physically and mentally demanding visit to Moscow, he became ill with a mysterious condition which baffled all the doctors he consulted. After exhaustive tests and two weeks in hospital he was at the point of death. A report left by one doctor for another and read by Cousins said: 'I'm afraid we may be losing Norman.' None of the consultants could give a precise diagnosis, although there was a consensus among them that he was suffering from a serious collagen illness - a disintegration of the connective tissue between the cells. For this they gave him two dozen aspirins a day, sleeping pills to sleep, and pain-relieving drugs. His own doctor told him he had only one chance in 500 of recovering from this mysterious condition.

It was at that point that Cousins took matters into his own hands. He sent for books on stress, and read: 'If negative emotions produce chemical changes, then positive emotions could produce positive changes.' Discharging himself from hospital and booking a hotel room, he sent for some Marx Brothers' movies and a film projector and took himself off all drugs. He says that every night he literally laughed himself to sleep. He sent for and took massive doses of vitamin C intravenously. He read many humorous books such as *The Enjoyment of Laughter*.

Writing his own account of the experience Cousins said:

> Two or three doctors have commented that I was probably the beneficiary of a mammoth venture in self-administered placebos. Such a hypothesis bothers me not at all. Respectable names in the history of medicine, like Paracelsus and Osler, have suggested that the history of medication is far more the history of the placebo effect than of intrinsically valuable and relevant drugs.[72]

UNNECESSARY DRUGS

The evidence shows that nature itself is the best healing process, with the doctor as the best healing agent - that is, the doctor as he or she was before aspirin was discovered in 1899 and rarely as he or she is today. In 1962, when the United States Food and Drug Administration examined the 4,300 prescription drugs that had appeared since World War II, only two out of five were found to be effective. A few years ago in Britain an official circular sent to all medical practitioners stated that after four months continuous use, Valium ceased to be effective and became addictive; yet tens of thousands of doctors continue to prescribe Valium regularly for their unwitting patients - many of whom are probably warning their teenage offspring about the dangers of becoming addicted to marijuana. To patients who regularly take Valium I say: 'Try coming off the drug for a few days and watch what happens; you will have all the symptoms of withdrawal.'

It has been estimated by experienced clinicians that between 20 to 50 drugs are all that will ever be needed for 98 per cent of the population. Dr Vernon Coleman, in his book, *The Medicine Men*, reports seven out of ten British doctors prescribe placebos for unhappiness, and quotes a statement that family doctors in Britain estimate that up to a third of their patients have nothing wrong with them and are simply unhappy.[63]

Dr Colin Brewer, writing in *World Medicine*, noted that, with the exception of schizophrenics, patients taking part in clinical trials of psychiatric drugs often respond in greater numbers to the placebo than specifically to the active drug. He commented that, in the relatively mild disorders which account for most psychiatric problems seen in general practice, it was common to find that 40 to 50 per cent of the patients responded to the placebo, and it was rare for the proportion who responded to the active drug to exceed this figure by more than 10 or 20 per cent. He added:

> We know, furthermore, that it is not even necessary to administer drugs to make patients feel better. A trial of dynamic psychotherapy versus behaviour therapy revealed that the control group, who merely had a thorough psychiatric history taken and were then placed on a waiting list, improved to the tune of 70 per cent; in many respects this was as good as the psychodynamic patients, and almost as good as the behavioural group.[40]

In a letter to the *British Medical Journal*, Dr J. Guy Edwards declared:

> In 15 studies involving 1082 patients with a wide variety of organic and psychiatric disorders placebos had an average significant effectiveness of 35.2 per cent and were most effective when stress was greatest. In the Medical Research Council's trial of the treatment of depressive illness about a third of the patients receiving placebo 'wholly or almost wholly lost their symptoms' within the first four weeks.[98]

This leaves many patients who would recover without the administration of drugs, but because of the withdrawal they experience when trying to stop these drugs, they think that the drugs are still necessary.

There is little doubt in my own mind that the placebo effect plays a significant role in substance abuse, as it does even in cancer, from whatever stimulus. In some ways still unknown to us, the brain is able to pick up a message which it then transforms by conviction into biochemical changes. And since there are stress factors involved in cancer and in substance abuse, the appropriate stimulus to effect amelioration of these stress factors is of critical importance. The 'appropriate stimulus', in medical terms, could be either electromagnetic or chemical, but in philosophical terms it is associated with information and the strength and quality of belief in the information, however it is communicated.

DOES NET DEPEND ON THE PLACEBO EFFECT?

Few patients who have requested NET believed that an electrical stimulus could deal with an obsession as powerful as heroin - or cigarettes. They had lost the ability to believe, and their willpower had been dissipated by years of self-indulgence. Placebo alone was insufficient to bridge the gap between belief and willpower.

In animal experiments, the placebo factor is eliminated. Rats and mice addicted to morphine suffer withdrawal symptoms similar to those of humans: electrostimulation through the rats' ears significantly relieved the symptoms of withdrawal in these animals.[54, 219, 340]

Thus it is clear to me that the successes of NET cannot be attributed only, or mainly, to the placebo effect.

> Mike, 36, had been mainlining 2 grams of heroin daily for eight years and often up to 10 grams a day when available. In addition, he was injecting methadone (Physeptone ampoules for intravenous use) 120 milligrams daily, and sometimes up to 500 milligrams a day (12 to 50 ampoules); up to 10 grams of cocaine daily, often 'freebasing' it, during the same period; and at night he took four tablets of Mandrax. Part of this huge drug intake was legally prescribed because he was a registered addict at a government drug dependency unit. All his superficial veins were thrombosed and unusable. For the eight months previous to the NET treatment he had been injecting drugs into his right femoral vein (in the groin) up to 15 times a day. This area was a mass of thickened scars. I personally witnessed him insert a needle easily and unerringly when he withdrew a blood sample for testing because the nurses could not obtain it from a vein. He stated categorically he had no withdrawal symptoms at all with NET, and that his only complaint was not having a full

night's sleep until the ninth night. The nursing staff reported he had no signs of withdrawal. His urine was checked at the end of the first week and was negative for all drugs.

In the past few years, in the field of alcoholism, interesting experiments have been carried out at a number of American universities in what one report called 'the Think Drink Effect'. For example, if a person thinks he is drinking alcohol but is really drinking only tonic he will exhibit the same sort of uninhibited behaviour that he would normally attribute to the effects of alcohol.[200]

The psychological rationale behind these experiments was that a drinker is expecting a high; because of past experience, when he drinks he has a combination of physical effects of the alcohol and psychological expectations about it. This is compared to the well-known Pavlovian reaction - a dog salivates at the sound of a bell associated with the smell and taste of food; so the experienced drinker may achieve a conditioned high when presented with the cue properties of a drink (appearance, smell and taste), even when the simulated drink contains no alcohol whatever.

One study of inexperienced drinkers, involving 1,500 students aged 12 to 19, showed that actual experience was not necessary to have expectations of a high, ranging from reduction of tension to social pleasure to alteration of behaviour.

In another study, 32 volunteers were divided into four groups: members of one group were told they were drinking alcohol but were actually drinking a non-alcohol beverage similar in taste and appearance; one group was told they were not drinking alcohol and they were not; one group was told they were not drinking alcohol but they were; one group was told they were drinking alcohol and they were. From the study it was concluded that people's beliefs about alcohol were just as important as other factors. However, alcohol expectation affected only social behaviours such as conversation, sexual arousal and aggressiveness, and did not affect such skills as driving.

In a report in *The Lancet*, a research group in California investigated the possibility that placebos might act by stimulating the release of endorphins, in which case the effect should be abolished by an antagonist such as naloxone which blocks opioid receptors. This hypothesis was tested with a number of dental patients, some on morphine and some on placebo. About 40 per cent of the patients given a placebo reported relief of their pain. However, when they were given naloxone as a second injection these patients said that the pain became worse. In contrast, naloxone made little or no difference to the patients who had not responded to the placebo. Also, when naloxone was given as the first injection it not only failed to relieve pain but also reduced the likelihood of a placebo response to later injections.[183] The science column of the London *Times* of 23 September 1978 reported on this:

> This evidence provides strong support for the theory that placebo effects are mediated through endorphins. If indeed that is the mechanism it would explain some of the similarities between placebos and narcotic drugs. Both become less effective with repeated use; there is a tendency for the dose needed to rise with time; and withdrawal symptoms may develop when the opiate or placebo is stopped.

So NET, by enabling the brain to produce endorphins naturally, may bridge the gap between drugs and placebos.

Chapter 4
NET as experienced by patients

Eric Clapton's experience

Early on in my research a close friend asked me if I would treat the British rock music star, Eric Clapton (in the 1960s and early 1970s huge placards at rock concerts declared 'Eric Clapton is God'), who was badly incapacitated because of heroin addiction. Known internationally as the greatest blues guitarist of his time, his ability to play or compose had virtually disappeared as his addiction had increased. At the time I was still using the first model of my stimulator, and tiny acupuncture needles, with intermittent treatments during the day and none in the night.

At first, I lived in Eric's home while treating him. This arrangement was unsatisfactory because I could not control the situation. For example, a close friend of Eric's, Joel, who had come to help out, confided that Eric was putting pressure on him to sell his last guitar to get money for heroin, and he found it difficult to refuse - although he was convinced that when Eric's last guitar was sold, he would commit suicide. Eric agreed to continue his treatment in our home in London - at that time, a flat in Harley Street where I had my consulting rooms.

We arrived there on a Friday and the first prototype of my own design of stimulator was awaiting me. It was large and cumbersome - 2 feet by 10 inches by 8 inches. Up to then, in his own home, Eric had used the crude Chinese stimulator which I had bought in Hong Kong. The new stimulator seemed almost immediately to have much better effect.

However, on the Saturday morning, Eric developed severe stomach cramps and diarrhoea, for which I gave all the standard medicines, but nothing brought relief. I was almost as distressed as he was, particularly because this was his 6th day without heroin, and such symptoms should not occur so late. At 6 o'clock that evening, Eric wearily said, 'You know, Meg, I haven't been feeling anything on the machine all day.' Quickly I put the machine on myself and found that I too could not feel any current. I traced a wire which had become disconnected, repaired it - and after half an hour of NET, Eric's symptoms disappeared without any further medication and did not return. Although I regretted his day of discomfort, to me it was a striking confirmation that it was, in fact, the NET which had prevented the withdrawal symptoms, since, unknown to us both, he had not received any current the whole day. An unintentional double-blind trial.

Within five weeks, Eric was not only off all drugs but also had more drive and energy than he had had for years. Within three months he was back on the world's stage 'playing better than ever before' according to music critics.

Afterwards he said: 'I wasn't actually looking for a cure ... It made me stop wanting to take smack.'

The Keith Richards saga

I have had some extraordinary experiences over the last few years but possibly the most difficult and bizarre of all was in 1977, four years after I had begun my research in London.

Early that year I received an urgent telephone call from Canada asking me if I would treat Keith Richards of the rock music group the Rolling Stones. There was nothing unusual about this, for I had already been approached about possible treatment for Keith, after treating Eric Clapton and others known to him. But this time, the circumstances in which I was being asked to treat him were unusual to the point of absurdity.

The newspapers had been full of an international scandal regarding Margaret Trudeau, wife of the then Canadian Prime Minister, who allegedly spent a night or more at the hotel in Canada where the Rolling Stones were performing. New headlines replaced those when police discovered so much heroin in Keith Richards's hotel room that he was arrested, not merely for possession but for trafficking in drugs. That offence carried with it the possibility of 20 years in prison. There was considerable panic in the Rolling Stones' organization at the thought of their top musical performer being removed suddenly and committed to prison, with the consequent break-up of the famous group and the potential loss of millions of dollars. It was an even greater shock to Keith, with his history of massive drug abuse and the expectation of having to go 'cold turkey' in prison.

The political complications associated with the Prime Minister's wife and her relationship with the Rolling Stones were superimposed on the political necessity for the authorities to be seen making a suitable example of the notorious rock star, Keith Richards. This made it more difficult than usual for me.

There were further complications. Because it was so politically sensitive, the conditions of Keith's bail required him to remain on the North American continent; and any attempt at treatment (with its implications of leniency) meant that the doctor involved in the treatment would have to be prepared to swear in court that he or she could cure addictions and give evidence in support of the claim. The Rolling Stones had not been able to find a physician in Canada or the United States who would accept Keith as a patient under such circumstances, so they telephoned me. Would I come to the United States and treat Keith there? I said I would.

I was able to find a clinic and two American colleagues willing to accept the difficult assignment, Dr Richard Corbett and Dr Joseph Winston. Dr Corbett, with much experience in treating drug addictions, was Medical Director of the Lakeland Drug Abuse Clinic, in New Jersey. However, because of the political nature of the case the American authorities required us to describe our treatment plan for prior approval. We drew up a medical treatment protocol, for six weeks of detoxification and convalescence, which was acceptable to the US Government. To avoid publicity, it was agreed that Keith should be treated privately in the nearby home of Shorty and Jean Yeaworth, film producer friends of ours.

Despite all the difficulties, the treatment was successful, and the protocol signed by the three doctors - Corbett, Winston and myself - was accepted by the Canadian courts as evidence of the success of Keith's treatment, and he was not sent to prison. And in Keith Richards's words:

> It's so simple it's not true ... It's a little metal box with leads that clip on to your ears and in two or three days - which is the worst period for kicking junk - in these seventy-two hours it leaves your system. Actually, you should be incredibly sick, but for some reason you're not. Why? I don't know, because all it is is a very simple, nine-volt, battery-run operation.

BBC films about NET

A couple of years before this incident, the BBC had shown a film on NET called 'Off the Hook', in 1975. This film had shown a registered addict (who was injecting black-market heroin as well as the Physeptone supplied by his drug dependency unit) being taken through his NET treatment, day by day. The BBC had insisted that I should allow the film to be shown even if the treatment was a failure and they would then try to analyse the causes of failure. The patient was treated in our home, because he could not afford the cost of a private clinic. It was a tremendous strain, both on the patient and on us as a family, living under the television cameras day after day, but when the film was shown, and the improvement in both the patient's physical condition and attitude dramatically obvious, it all seemed worthwhile.

Two years later, the BBC did a follow-up film of the same addict. He looked well, was still off all drugs, and in full-time work. He lived alone in a flat in the worst area of London for drug-dealing. When the interviewer asked him why he had returned to a situation where he was surrounded by temptation, he pondered the question for a few moments and then replied, 'Because I knew if I couldn't return and survive here, I wasn't cured.' That was 1977, and in 1985 he remains well, busy, happily married and has a child.

The second film concluded with a segment filmed in the United States, in which Dr Corbett, one of the American doctors involved in the treatment of Keith Richards, was interviewed about his conclusions regarding NET. He said he was so impressed with its results that he was trying to persuade the US authorities to invite me to the United States.

In 1980 the BBC asked permission to make a third film about our work, concentrating partly on our clinic instead of one individual, and partly on the scientific rationale behind NET. They also interviewed several independent scientists for their opinion on NET, including one of the discoverers of endorphins. Even the scientists expressed cautious optimism, particularly since the beneficial effects of electrical stimulation in pain conditions were, by then, well established.

Patients were interviewed both during and after their NET treatment. A 60-year-old alcoholic businessman commented, 'I was so bad, I don't even remember coming into the clinic. It certainly is a much kinder treatment than the usual treatment with pills. I had no withdrawal symptoms except for some evening sweats. I felt no craving for alcohol at all.' A 20-year-old heroin addict said, 'This is the first time I have felt well since I started taking heroin three years ago. On heroin, you either don't feel or you feel awful ... But I feel empty. As Meg said, it's like losing your husband or your wife.' When the interviewer asked him if he thought the good results could be due to a placebo effect, he replied, 'Perhaps. But if it is placebo, it works!'

Pete Townshend on the 'black box'

In an accompanying interview to the article in *Omni* magazine (see pages 61–72), Pete Townshend gave his impressions of NET, both as used on himself and as he had seen it in the operative treatment of others in the previous eight years. Pete had first seen NET when he visited Eric Clapton during his treatment, and was so impressed that over the next few years he and his rock group The Who raised many thousands of pounds to help me with my research.

> The Who guitarist Pete Townshend traces his downward slide toward drugged oblivion to the troubled spring of 1980. Long months of touring had brought him to the brink of a marital rift. Gross financial mismanagement had left him $1 million in debt to English banks. And all the while he brooded incessantly about the future of The Who. 'I started drinking about a bottle and a half of cognac a day,' Townshend recalls. 'And to cut through the drunken stupor I was in, I got into this deadly alcohol-cocaine oscillation. Eventually I became such a physical wreck that I went to this doctor, who prescribed me sleeping pills and an anti-depressant (sic) called Ativan. These Ativans made me feel great, and soon I was taking eight to ten tablets a day, plus three sleeping pills every night. By Christmas, though, the Ativan stopped working, and so I turned to heroin. A month later it dawned on me that I was actually dying, that my macho "I-can-do-anything" mentality would kill me. It was then I contacted Meg.
>
> 'Even though I'd seen startling successes with her technique, I didn't know whether it would work for me. But by the second day I knew I was on the home straight. And on the third day I felt feelings of sexual desire returning, feelings of just wanting to go for a walk. It was incredible! There was a sense of inner joy as I started to gain independence from drugs. A natural energy flow slowly returned to my body. I could feel the old me coming back, and the first emotion I felt was arrogance. I thought, "This will be easy. A

few more days on this machine, and then I'll shoot up to L.A. and go dancing." That was my frame of mind. But the fourth day I got depressed. Initially I had been given low frequencies for heroin, but when I became depressed, I was given some high frequencies for my cocaine addiction. And at this high setting, I would sometimes have psychedelic experiences. The colours in the room would suddenly start to go wooo. Then I had another setback, followed by a day when I felt superhuman. It was just like being on heroin. But the next day I again felt like death warmed over. Some withdrawal symptoms even returned.

'Gradually, though, your mood levels off so that by the tenth day you feel fairly normal. In retrospect, I realize that the treatment is an education in itself. NET reeducates the brain to produce its own drugs, and in the process you learn something about your human potential. You come to realize that somewhere within you is the power to deal with crises, tensions and frustrations. So the treatment reaffirms one's faith in the self-healing process.

'Of course it seems incredibly crude to shoot a thousand-cycle pulse through the brain – and *voilà!* Yet that's the beauty of it. There's something almost mystical about recovering by such a ridiculously simple technique. Somehow a simple little gadget has made me feel whole. And if I'm ever raped by a crazed pusher and become hooked all over again, I won't hesitate to call Meg and have my addiction handled in this straightforward completely technical way.'[226]

These are well-known public figures who have spoken to the media on many occasions about their addictions and treatment by NET; there is thus no breach of medical ethics in using their names.

Addicts treated with NET by other doctors

The following are examples from the *Omni* article, of patients treated by a team who were trained by me, even though I myself did not participate in the treatment.

Stuart Harris started shooting heroin as a 16-year-old cadet in the Royal Navy. By the time he underwent NET in the spring of 1981, he had been addicted to heroin for 15 years, and for 11 of those years he had also injected methadone intravenously. 'I had the sweats very badly,' he says of his experience on NET. 'You're emitting all this bad grunge from your body, and you feel you're speeding (on amphetamines). But there's no withdrawal at all. That much I'll say for it. I mean when they told me about it, I just took it with a pinch of salt - another treatment they've fobbed off on the poor junkies. But, believe me, if I was getting any pain as I used to have with withdrawals, I wouldn't have stayed there, 'cause I was a voluntary patient. When I discharged myself from hospital, I didn't go searching for drugs as I would normally have done in the past, say, after methadone reduction or narcosis (that's when they sedate you up to your eyeballs in sleeping pills). After completing all the other methods, I felt so uptight all the time. The first thing I wanted to do was have a massive great fix. But, after NET, all you really want to do is sleep. Everything is so easygoing. I can't say that it (heroin) doesn't drift into my mind. Like the other day, I fancied a fix. But it passed over in a few minutes. Before, if I'd felt the slightest urge for a fix, off I'd go to London. Something has changed. You feel calmer. You can accept the ups and downs.'

A 28-year-old man, who requested anonymity, combined a high level of alcohol and marijuana consumption with a cocaine habit of two to six grams each week for more than seven years (the cocaine alone usually cost him more than $1,000 a month). He agreed to speak to *Omni* immediately after completing NET treatment in the summer of 1982. 'Until this therapy,' he says, 'I couldn't go three days without feeling an enormous craving for drugs. Cocaine and, to a lesser degree, alcohol would always be on my mind. But from the moment the electrodes were put on my head, my craving immediately diminished. When I had passed the three-day mark, I felt no craving at all, and I still don't. Drugs never enter my mind. Now that I remember what it's like to feel good - to be clearheaded after all these years - I'm certain that I won't go back on drugs.'

Rachel Waite, a heavy smoker for five years, was treated for her cigarette addiction in June 1981. 'For the first three days on NET,' she recalls, 'I still had the urge to smoke, and I probably would have lit up had a cigarette been handy. However, by the end of treatment I definitely did not want one. When I took an experimental puff, it was a different sensation altogether. It tasted foul, and there was no hit whatsoever. It was as if I was drawing on hot air.'

Long-term follow up

In a seven-year follow-up statistical survey of 186 addicts treated by NET from 1973 to December 1980 (130 on drugs, 30 on alcohol, 26 on cigarettes) partly funded by the British Medical Association and which I completed recently,[242] it was demonstrated that

78.5 per cent of those who were traced at follow-up were drug, alcohol, and cigarette-free; for drug-use only, 80 per cent.

Cigarettes are a harder addiction than heroin to stop, but methadone is the hardest of all to discontinue. However, the most severe and prolonged withdrawal symptoms are produced by tranquillizers such as Ativan and Valium, that is without NET. Many users now report persistent symptoms for up to 2 years after stopping tranquillizers, and documented reports have been published in journals such as the *British Medical Journal.*[21]

In addition, only 23 per cent of NET patients made alcohol a substitute dependence, and all of these temporarily. This is compared with other programmes where 60 per cent of addicts treated became moderate or 'heavy' drinkers. Sixty-five per cent of those who were drug and alcohol free, after the 10 days of NET, had no 'rehabilitation' at all or less than 14 days.

The drop-out rate for all patients who began NET over the seven years was 1.6 per cent. This compared with published figures in the UK and USA of other treatment modalities which reflected a 45 to 90 per cent drop-out rate.[152, 286, 324] Fifty-nine per cent of the addicts treated (including the alcohol and cigarette figures) were under 30 years of age. The average length of stay in 'rehabilitation' for all NET patients was 16 days. In other programmes 'success' depended on the length of time in the programme, usually 18 months or longer.

My lowest success rate has been with smoking (44 per cent still cigarette free at follow-up), yet the Research Committee of the British Thoracic Society reported in 1983 that comparing four methods of smoking withdrawal for 1,550 patients, only 9.7 per cent had successfully stopped smoking at the end of a year.[260] Although there have been various claims for the effectiveness of nicotine chewing gum as an aid to stopping smoking, this study did not result in greater success when either nicotine or placebo chewing gum was used to reinforce verbal advice.

In another controlled trial of nicotine chewing gum, conducted in general practice, of the 200 participants 99 were given placebo gum. When assessed after six months, only 18 of the 200 had been successful in stopping smoking; of these, 10 were on active gum and 8 on placebo.[154] Moreover, the nicotine gum may itself be addictive.[284]

IMMEDIATE EFFECTS OF NET

Although NET can be used either in an inpatient or outpatient setting (the stimulator is pocket-size and the patient is completely mobile throughout the 10-day treatment), the first follow-up of NET patients[238] showed that long-term outcomes are considerably better for inpatients. Unless the patient has a supportive family or community who are able to give constant supervision, he is likely to use drugs or alcohol during treatment; the clinical evidence is that concomitant drug use slows down the beneficial effects of NET. (It may, in fact, produce severe aversive effects, particularly in cocaine use.)

Even nicotine addicts find three to four days of inpatient treatment preferable, because it is easier for them to stop their cigarettes totally when away from the stresses of daily life.

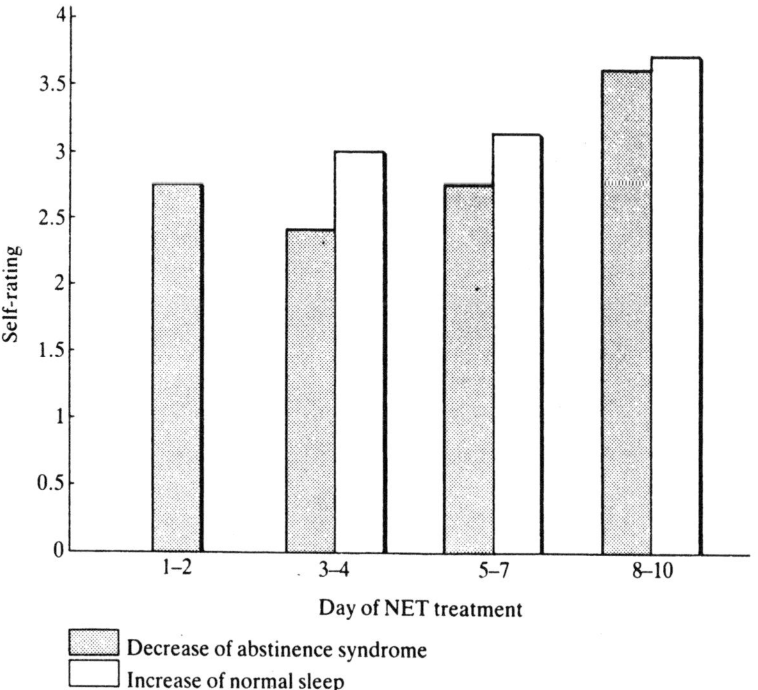

Figure 4.1 Quality of physical condition (as measured by the abstinence syndrome) and of natural sleep, both as estimated by the patients themselves. O indicates the worst condition and 4 the best. The ratings by the nursing staff were only minimally higher than the ratings by the patients. $n = 102$.

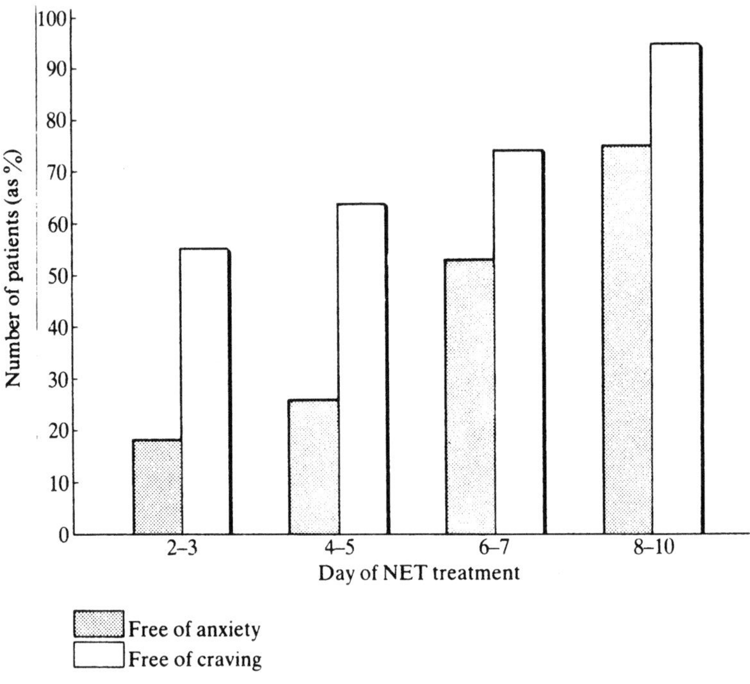

Figure 4.2 Total number of patients per day reporting freedom from anxiety and from craving. $n = 101$ for days 2 to 5; $n = 95$ for days 6 to 10 (cigarette patients required only five days of NET).

Figures 4.1 and 4.2 (see also Figures 8.1, 8.2 and 8.3 on pages 153-55) show the overall effects of NET on the acute abstinence syndrome, as computerized from the Clinic charts of patients treated from January to December, 1980.

Figure 4.1 shows the minimum withdrawal symptoms experienced under NET, by the patients' own estimates - and that is with no replacement drugs whatever. It also illustrates the rapid return of natural sleep, instead of the weeks or even months of insomnia following any other method of withdrawal.

Craving, anxiety and lethargy are common to withdrawal from all psychoactive drugs, and persist for many months. Figure 4.2 shows how rapidly the craving and anxiety are reduced within the 10 days of NET.

PATIENTS' PROGRESS

The following is a summary of the progress of patients treated with NET in England from October 1973 to December 1980.

1 *Type of addiction*

There were 186 patients with the following main addictions:

drugs (legal and illegal	130
alcohol	30
cigarettes	26

(Note: Patients treated by NET for conditions other than the above are *not* included in this survey.)

2 *Years of using the addictive substance daily*

0.5-1 year	8%
2-4 years	30%
5-10 years	40%
11-20 years	15%
21-30 years	4%
Over 30 years	3%

(Majority of drug addicts were main-liners who injected the drug into a vein.)

3 *Amount of daily drug use on admission for NET*

Slight (within the maximum recommended limit for drugs)	23%
Moderate	37%
Heavy	26%
Extremely heavy	14%

These daily amounts ranged from 300 mg prescribed heroin to 10 g street heroin (officially up to 40 per cent purity in London in 1980); cocaine 0.5-10 g; methadone 40-800 mg. Various narcotic or psychotropic drugs up to 70 tablets daily. (*All* drugs were stopped totally and immediately on commencing NET.)

4 *Patient drop-out rate*

Patient drop-out rate over seven years of those who began NET but did not complete five days of detoxification was 1.6 per cent. (Compare with published figures in UK and USA of other treatments modalities of from 45 per cent to 75 per cent to 90 per cent drop-out rate.)

5 *Follow-up of patients*

Summary of information received from postal questionnaires (multiple outcome variables) or direct reporting for NET follow-up one to eight years after treatment, with a return rate of 50 per cent (see Figure 4.3).

> 80 per cent were drug free. (Others have been reported drug free since the review was completed.)
> 78 per cent were alcohol free. (An additional seven alcoholics whose goal on admission was controlled drinking all reported success.) 44 per cent were cigarette free.
> (USA figures indicate that 'when effectiveness is defined in terms

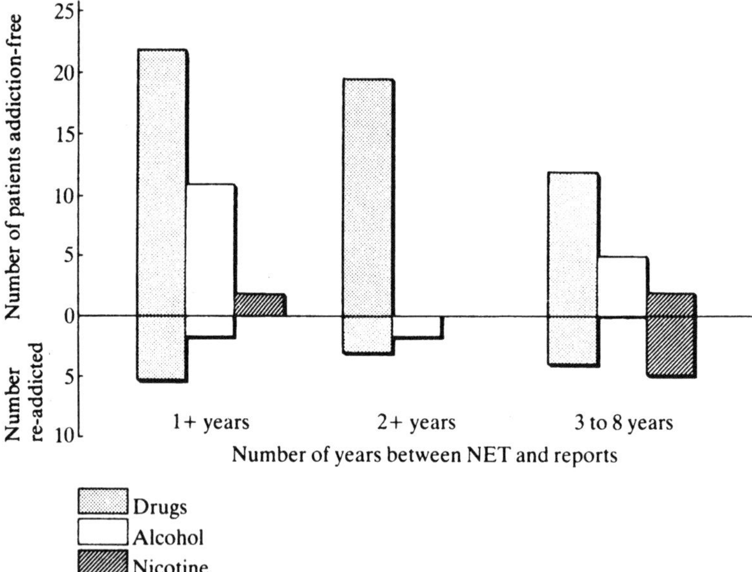

Figure 4.3 Follow-up of patients treated by NET for drug, alcohol and nicotine addictions from 1973 to December 1980. Of treated patients, 50 per cent were traced, out of a total of 186 to whom questionnaires were sent. The poorest response rate was from smokers (35 per cent). The upper half of the chart represents the addiction-free patients, the lower half of the chart those who were re-addicted at the time of the follow-up.

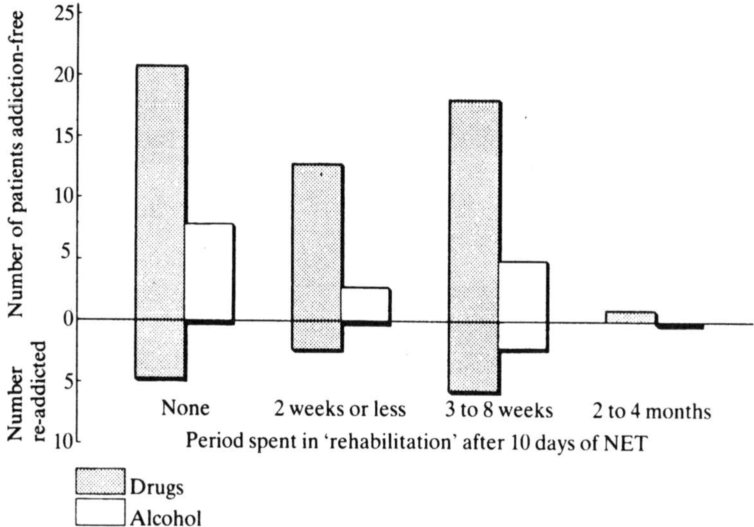

Figure 4.4 Relationship between time spent in 'rehabilitation' after completion of 10 days of NET, and long-term outcome. Statistically, the long-term outcome appears to be unaffected by the length of time spent in some kind of institution after completion of NET. However, a short period of intensive 'rehabilitation' may be of value to some, depending on individual character and needs. Both individual and group counselling is given during the 10 days of NET.

of heroin or methadone abstinence, *less than 10 per cent* are judged successful 10 years after treatment.')

60 per cent were less than 30 years old.

65 per cent had less than two weeks or no 'rehabilitation' at all after their ten days of NET; the average length of stay in 'rehab' for all NET patients was *16 days* (see Figure 4.4). (In other programmes, 'success' depended on the length of time in the programme, usually *18 months* or longer.)

67 per cent reported decreased use of alcohol, cigarettes and/or marijuana.

75 per cent reported improved sleep.

87 per cent reported improved health.

77 per cent had never made alcohol a substitute dependence.

23 per cent had temporarily made alcohol a substitute dependence (though drug-free).

0 per cent were dependent on alcohol at the time of the questionnaire. (Compare USA government figures published in 1982;

60 per cent of those treated became heavy or very heavy drinkers.)
68 per cent rarely feel a craving for the drug, alcohol, or cigarette (though drug-free).
15 per cent occasionally feel a craving for the drug, alcohol, or cigarette (though drug-free).
17 per cent frequently feel a craving for the drug, alcohol, or cigarette (though drug-free).

6 *Statistical report of the 21.5 per cent who became re-addicted*

78 per cent were using less of their substance of abuse than before NET.
44 per cent reported improved health.
64 per cent reported improved relationships with spouse/family.
50 per cent were more able to cope with daily problems.

All drug addicts, including the recidivists, had diminished their alcohol intake.

CONCLUSIONS

The foregoing statistics provide the necessary skeletal framework of our approach to the problem of addiction. To transform this into a dynamic structure required a lot more official support. Friends and colleagues concerned to help with the worldwide problem were urging relevant departments and governments to take note of this research.

'Meg Patterson has now devoted many years to refining her NeuroElectric method of treatment. I have seen it work, and I believe it should play an important role in the strategy of all governments, who are wrestling with the drug problem.' These words were written by the late the Rt Hon. Lord Harlech, former British Ambassador to the USA. A *centrally-funded* residential clinic or clinics, medically staffed, could provide the 10 days detoxification, and then return the patients to their local health authority to provide an on-going 'support system'.

The cost-effectiveness is obvious. Instead of supplying addicts with drugs and sterile syringes every day for 10, perhaps 20 years, which is the main function of most drug dependency units, the NET costs would only be the staffing of such clinics, the addicts' train fares, and the initial purchase of NET stimulators. It has been my experience that not many addicts are willing to accept 18 months (the usual practice) in a residential 'rehabilitation' centre, but probably many would be prepared to stay for up to two months. The clinical evidence (see above description of the seven-year follow-up of NET treated addicts) is that about two months of rehabilitation following on NET is as effective as 18 months after the usual withdrawal methods, or even more so, because of the seeming elimination of the symptoms of chronic withdrawal.

The MEGNET stimulator is not itself addictive. After 10 days of treatment, it had completed its work, no matter how large the dosage, the type of drug, or the duration of drug usage.

There would still be recidivists, but for a considerable number the relapse or relapses would be only temporary and no further active treatment would be required. But for those who do require another 10-day treatment, that would still cost less than either drug-maintenance or long-term residential rehabilitation. It would be essential to have sufficient beds available to eliminate the present long waiting-lists; as with the City Road's Drug Crisis Centre in London, there must always be room for the hospital patient recovering from an overdose of drugs of addiction, or even for the addict who suddenly decides that 'now is the time to stop'.

As Sir Yehudi Menuhin, the internationally famous violinist, says, 'Only public and governmental lethargy and blind exploitation of pain and misery stand in the way of Dr Patterson's approach - as spiritual as it is psychological, as rational as it is compassionate. As with the greatest advances in knowledge, this overwhelming advance can reverse the lamentable trend of our civilization, by a process of healing, of health, and of hope.' NET will not stop people from experimenting with or abusing drugs: it does offer a way out of the prison which drug abusers have entered.

II SCIENTIFIC RATIONALE AND RESULTS

Chapter 5
Hong Kong: Surgery, serendipity and stimulation

Acupuncture

I first became interested in acupuncture in England in 1963, when my husband George, a journalist, was assisting a senior colleague with the London *Observer*, Guy Wint, to edit a book on Asian affairs.[347] At that time Guy suffered a severe stroke which left him partially paralysed and with impaired speech. Reduced to frustrating inactivity, he also suffered continuous pain requiring heavy sedation. Guy heard of Dr Felix Mann, a consultant in my old hospital, St James's, Balham, who practised acupuncture. At Guy's request I discussed the treatment with Dr Mann. A few years later in *The Third Killer*, Guy described his experience of a variety of treatments in different parts of the world:

> By far the most rewarding of these experiments was with Chinese acupuncture. It was surprising that this was so because at first the doctor who practised it - Dr Felix Mann from Cambridge, trained in Western medicine - asserted that it would do little for strokes, and tried to dissuade me from having this administration. Later I discovered in a Chinese handbook that the Chinese themselves use it in such cases, but they recognize that a stroke is altogether a very serious matter, and a cure is not very likely.[348]

I was so impressed by Guy's improvement, and by that of several others whom I sent to Dr Mann for treatment, that when I arrived in Hong Kong in September 1964 I decided to have acupuncture treatment for my own migraine headaches. I had suffered from migraine for 30 years, with three three-day attacks almost every two weeks, made tolerable only by large doses of pain-relieving drugs.

I was introduced by a mutual friend to a Chinese acupuncturist. He was a film distributor, not a doctor, but he had studied and practised acupuncture all his life, first in China and later in France, and was well-informed on the subject of human anatomy. He recommended three courses of treatment over a period of three months.

The first month's treatments were dramatically successful. Both the frequency and intensity of the migraine attacks were reduced by 95 per cent. In the second month, with the needles placed in the corner of my eye in addition to other sites, improvement was only 50 per cent. In the third month, the attacks were as severe as ever and the needling, which was at first painless, became very painful. I discontinued the treatment.

The same acupuncturist later treated my husband successfully for an arthritic knee stemming from a damaged cartilage, the legacy of an old football injury, which began to be very painful and caused George sleepless nights. I arranged an appointment with an orthopaedic surgeon colleague, who established by X-ray that there were osteoarthritic changes in the knee and gave George cortisone injections. Six weeks later the pain was back, as unbearable as ever. However, after two half-hour treatments with needles and electrical stimulation by the acupuncturist the pain disappeared and did not return.

ELECTRO-ACUPUNCTURE

One of my Chinese colleagues in the 850-bed Tung Wah Hospital, where I was head of surgery, was Dr H. L. Wen, a well-known Hong Kong neurosurgeon, who was consultant to the neurosurgical unit. Dr Wen became extremely interested in the possibilities of using acupuncture anaesthesia for some of his brain operations. After six weeks' visit in China to study the technique, he returned to Hong Kong and asked me to select some patients who were willing to have electro-acupuncture anaesthesia for their operations instead of orthodox anaesthesia. Another colleague involved in the experiments was Dr Wen's senior assistant, Dr Stanley Y.C. Cheung, one of my own trainee surgeons who had assisted me before sitting for his Edinburgh Fellowship and doing further advanced training at the Edinburgh neurosurgical unit.

Various forms of stimulation are used by the Chinese in addition to the common needle and finger acupuncture. In injection acupuncture, sterile water, saline, morphine, etc., are injected into acupuncture points. In thread acupuncture, catgut threaded to a surgical needle is passed from one acupuncture point to another. In pressure acupuncture pressure is applied to the skin over the acupuncture points.

Stimulation is achieved either manually, through a push-pull or rotary movement, or by a regulatory current in the case of electro-acupuncture. Manual stimulation is carried out for 10 to 15 minutes and the needle either removed or left in place until the next session, when the procedure is repeated.

Electro-acupuncture stimulation, with the stimulator attached to the acupuncture needles, gained widespread use in acupuncture anaesthesia during the 1950s because it produces continued stimulation over longer periods of time with much less effort on the part of the operator. Also, the strength of the stimulation can be adjusted according to the needs of the patient, and a stronger stimulation may be achieved than with the manual rotation of the needles.

Drs Wen, Cheung and I started experimenting with the 6.26 stimulator which was widely used in China, and had a bipolar spike wave form, AC current, pulse width 0.6 msec and a frequency up to 111 hertz (Hz, cycles per second).

AN UNEXPECTED DISCOVERY

While producing acupuncture analgesia by this machine, we made an unexpected discovery. In a remarkable example of serendipity we found that we were also curing drug addicts. Unknown to us, some of our patients had been on drugs - opium, heroin, morphine - for a number of years. Some had been heavily addicted for many years to doses far in excess of anything tolerated in the West. They volunteered the information spontaneously, that, within a few days after we started needling them they had, for the first time, lost their desire for drugs.

It was Dr Wen who first suggested a possible connection between acupunctural stimulation operating on the autonomic nervous system, and the withdrawal symptoms of drug addiction. He then asked me to select a wider range of drug addicts from among the hospital patients, or from the sophisticated young addicts who, I had told him, came to our home seeking help. We began to keep a detailed record of their responses, with increasing interest.

In February 1973, a well-known American neurosurgeon and neurophysiologist, Dr S. Irving Cooper, visited Hong Kong and gave a lecture to the Tung Wah Hospital staff. Dr Cooper, of St

Barnabas Hospital for Nervous Diseases in New York, became internationally known as a pioneer of several new brain operations for involuntary movement disorders (including Parkinson's disease) and for techniques in cryogenic surgery. At his lecture Dr Cooper revealed that he had discovered a possible means of curing spastics and epileptics by surgically implanting electrodes in the patients' brains and then stimulating them by means of a receiver implanted in the chest, activated by a pocket transmitter. His theory was that prosthetic stimulation of the cerebellum may gradually recondition reflex functioning of some brain circuits or lead to enduring neurochemical changes.[67]

These findings were deeply challenging to me. If some connection could be established between what Dr Cooper was investigating, and our own discovery of the effects of electrically stimulated acupuncture, some tremendous possibilities might be developed. Dr Cooper himself was very interested when I raised the subject with him at a private meeting a few days later. He affirmed that some present theories about brain physiology might have to be reconsidered in the light of such developments. He added that recent neurosurgical evidence suggested that electrical stimulation reconditioned circuits such as the reticular formation, so that in conditions formerly considered incurable there was progressive improvement the longer the treatment was carried on.

Later, on reflection, an idea suddenly struck me: what if the Chinese, without knowing about electricity, had stumbled, several thousand years before, on another profound discovery? Acupuncture might well be a form of electrical stimulation to correct a metabolic imbalance; the recent electro-acupuncture stimulation might be simply eliciting a more intense form of the response than the original twirling practice. If so, in the drug addiction cures we had witnessed, the precise acupuncture points would be less important than general electrical stimulation of the nerve pathways to the brain - occurring in some way yet to be identified.

To follow up these and other ideas that were emerging from our researches, I expanded my reading into the new fields of acupuncture and electrical stimulation, in Western as well as Chinese literature, to uncover any connection between electrical stimulation and drug addictions. I already knew from my own reading that electro-convulsive therapy (shock treatment) had been used in alcoholism and other addictions with marked lack of success. Somewhere between that failure and our recent successful experience with the much milder electro-acupuncture, I suspected I would find an answer.

Chinese medicine

Chinese herbal medicine is over 4,000 years old. The first pharmacy book, the *P'en T'sao*, published by the Emperor Shen Nung in 2737 BC, listed 365 herbs as superior, mediocre or inferior. The now famous ephedrine, brought to the notice of the West by a Dr K. K. Chen in 1926, was listed in the *P'en T'sao* as *ma huang*, and had been used by Chinese doctors to treat asthma for 4,000 years.

The *Huang Ti Nei Ching Su Wen* or *The Yellow Emperor's Classic of Internal Medicine* is the earliest extant medical classic of China. Written between the eighth and fifth centuries BC it consists of 18 volumes covering a great variety of subjects, including the theory of diseases and their aetiology, diagnosis and treatment.

In the book, man is seen as a microcosm of the universe, subject to the same tensions as nature itself. The immutable course of nature, the *tao*, was believed to act through two opposing and unifying forces, the *yin* (negative, passive and feminine) and the *yang* (positive, active and masculine). In a normal person the two forces are in balance and assist the vital energy (called *chi*) to circulate to all parts of the body via a network of 14 channels, or 'meridians', each connected to an important internal organ or junction to which it branches. Obstruction (deficiency) and outpouring (excess) in the circulation of the *chi* causes an imbalance of the two forces, and thus results in disease.

Traditional Chinese medicine and philosophy were based on this concept of *chi*. It was believed that all things, animate or inanimate, possessed an inherent energy. This energy stabilized the chemical composition of matter, and when this matter was broken down energy was released. Water and ice have the same chemical formula, yet when ice changes into water, energy in some form is released. Man is made of matter, but he has life also. Thus he has two sources of energy: the electrical energy generated as a result of biochemical and biophysical changes in his cells; and the living energy inherited by his birth. Dr Louis Moss, a Western expert on acupuncture, has stated: 'It may well be that this force (*chi*) is an electrical potential emanating from the minutest cells in the body by their biochemical and biophysical exchanges.'

The Chinese phrase for medicine consists of four radicals, or symbols, in two characters, one meaning a cavity with an arrow inside it, and the other meaning a knife or instrument and alcohol. Chinese scholars interpret the phrase to mean that an arrow has created a wound and that a knife or some other instrument is needed to extract it, with alcohol applied to treat it. So, in spite of later speculations and often absurd theories as to the causation and cure of diseases, among Chinese medical practitioners a rational, semi-scientific and dignified practice of empirical treatment has always existed, based on the accumulated knowledge of centuries and derived from acute observation by practitioners of intelligence and integrity.

Acupuncture (from the Latin *acus*, meaning 'needle', and *pungere*, meaning 'sting') has been used in China, some claim, for almost 5,000 years. However the practice of acupuncture developed in conjunction with 'moxibustion' or the burning of the herb *mugwort* at or near appropriate sites of the body. Thus the Chinese name for acupuncture, *chen-chiu*, meaning 'needle and heat', usually implies both practices. Acupuncture and moxibustion, combined with the use of herbs, breathing exercises, and therapeutic massage, still constitute the core of traditional Chinese medicine.

WESTERN MEDICINE IN CHINA

Before the West, with its recently developed system of scientific medicine, made an impact on China, the health of the nation depended on the practitioners of this traditional form of Chinese medicine. The Chinese doctor rarely practised surgery and, under the Manchu dynasty, from the 17th century to early in the 20th, he was not allowed to do so.

With the introduction of Western medicine in China, traditional Chinese medicine in general and acupuncture in particular began to fall into disrepute as being non-scientific. In 1822, after the official 'Great Imperial Board' in Peking ordered a virtual abandonment of acupuncture, Chinese intellectuals educated in Western missionary schools came to regard Chinese medicine as old-fashioned and a hindrance to the modernization and development of their country. In 1929 the Nationalist government banned the practice of traditional Chinese medicine, including acupuncture.

Despite such official opposition, the ordinary Chinese citizen continued to believe in and use acupuncture and traditional medicine. The 80 per cent of the population living in rural areas received virtually no benefit from the Western-trained doctors in the cities, and they continued to use herbal medicines and acupuncture for the relief of pain and various diseases.

Then the Communist government, after taking office in 1949, introduced the policy of 'walking on both feet', or using the best of both Chinese and Western medicine. Chairman Mao Zedong set out four concepts of health care: to serve the workers, peasants and soldiers; to put prevention first; to unite Western and traditional Chinese medicine; and to coordinate medical campaigns with mass movements. This policy gave rise to the mass medical phenomenon of 'barefoot doctors', personnel given some basic training, who went into the villages, towns, and cities to treat the people.

CHINA'S DOOR OPENS

In 1972 President Richard Nixon made his momentous visit to China, accompanied by a large entourage of journalists and doctors. The door into China which this visit opened to the West provided a fascinating variety of political opportunities and significant medical and scientific exchanges. For example, newspaper reports which flooded out of China during the presidential visit were filled with spectacular accounts of surgical operations being conducted by means of electro-acupuncture analgesia.

Shortly after his arrival in Beijing (Peking) with the presidential party, *New York Times* columnist James Reston developed appendicitis. His appendix was removed under conventional anaesthesia by surgeons at the Anti-Imperial Hospital in Beijing, but afterwards he permitted an acupuncturist to apply needles to his elbow and legs to relieve post-surgical pain. Reston wrote: 'There was a noticeable relaxation of pressure and distension within an hour, and no recurrence of the problem, thereafter.'

USA physicians soon began taking acupuncture seriously, especially when a group of their most eminent colleagues, including Boston heart specialist Dr Paul Dudley White and New York ear surgeon Dr Samuel Rosen, toured Chinese hospitals and watched fully conscious patients undergo major surgery with nothing more than acupuncture needles to anaesthetize them. The operations observed by the astonished doctors included partial removal of the stomach, excision of a brain tumour, and removal of an ovarian cyst. On his return to the USA Dr Rosen reported: 'My colleagues and I have seen the past, and it works.'

Other doctors visiting China were equally impressed by developments in Chinese medicine. Dr E. Grey Dimond, provost of the

University of Missouri Medical School in Kansas City, was one. In the *Journal of the American Medical Association* he cited advantages the Chinese had found in acupuncture anaesthesia: 'It is absolutely safe; there is no interruption of the patient's hydration. The patient can still receive fluid and food. There is no post-operative nausea and vomiting. The method is convenient and readily available.'

What happens in acupuncture?

Chinese doctors told their Western colleagues they used electro-acupuncture anaesthesia simply because it worked. Despite its use on over 500,000 patients with a 90 per cent success rate,[1] they could still offer no adequate explanation of its rationale. The leading theory inside China was that acupuncture as an anaesthetic involved 'neuro-physiological phenomena, and that basically the twirling needles were thought to send an impulse to the brain that reduced the electrical activity there which would otherwise register pain'.

The most widely accepted theory in the 1970s of how acupuncture works was that the prick of a needle at certain precisely defined points on the skin stimulates specific nerves which transmit electrical impulses via the spinal cord and lower centres of the brain, which in turn controls the affected area. Every part of the body, no matter how small, is supplied with nerves, and every millimetre of it is under the direct control of one nerve or group of nerves. Nerves control nearly all processes going on in the body. When stimulated, some nerves, for example, increase the movement of the intestines while others retard it; some increase, others retard, the flow of digestive juices. Similarly, certain nerves can increase or decrease the rate of the heartbeat, determine the expansion or contraction of blood vessels, and so on.

Dr Felix Mann has written:

> The nervous system can be compared to the electronic control apparatus of some complex machine, like a telephone exchange or an automatic pilot. The art of acupuncture depends on knowing precisely which nerve to stimulate in a given disease. It sounds as simple as knowing which keys to press on a typewriter in order to spell your name. In fact, however, a considerable amount of knowledge is necessary before acupuncture can be practised satisfactorily.[198]

Contemporary theories have now, of course, expanded to absorb the discovery of the endorphins and other naturally occurring substances (see pages 126–28).

ACUPUNCTURE ANAESTHESIA

Acupuncture was first used for surgical anaesthesia (the correct term is analgesia) in China in 1958. The first successful application was for tonsillectomy. Previously, following tonsillectomy under the usual local anaesthesia, the patient complained of sore throat and inability to eat or drink for several days. Since acupuncture was noted to be effective in relieving sore throat and pharyngitis it was first proposed that the procedure should be used for post-operative sore throat; finally acupuncture was combined with the anaesthesia procedure for the whole tonsillectomy, with great success.

The first experiments recorded by the Chinese were carried out on 660 medical personnel and other volunteers, followed by 40,000 other trial cases over the next few years. From these investigations psychiatrists began to experiment with possible new methods of treatment for psychiatric diseases, on the theory that it should be possible to transmit electricity through the sensory nerves to the higher centres of the brain without adversely affecting the motor cortex, as happens in electric shock treatment.

Traditionally, psychiatric treatment aimed at inhibiting the activities of the cerebrum, with physiological as well as pathological symptoms being suppressed. When acupuncture – using the electrical stimulation – was tried, it appeared to suppress only the pathological activities, leaving the physiological activities of the cerebrum intact. In studies at the Shanghai Psychiatric Hospital, 73 per cent of the patients treated showed good to fair response.[186]

One patient in a catatonic stupor lay completely motionless in bed, and did not eat, drink or utter a word. His dependence on others was total. Previously, the only treatment for this condition had been electric shock therapy, but the relapse rate was always high. After several electrical stimulations of his acupuncture points, the patient gradually recovered, not only eating and drinking normally but also talking rationally.

The investigators considered their application of electro-acupuncture through the trigeminal nerve to be analogous to the evolution of external to internal pacemakers for heart stimulation. In order to overcome the impedance of the skin and chest wall, the external pacemaker needed a current of 60 to 70 volts and caused annoying stimulation of the chest muscles. The internal pacemaker, with the tip of the electrode in the right ventricular wall, needed a current of only one millivolt, and did not stimulate any surrounding structures.

Experiments were conducted on animals as well as humans. Sensitive electronic instruments were attached to the brain, and the electric activity of the brain recorded. Stimulation of the trigeminal nerve elicited the strongest and widest distribution of the electric waves. On the other hand, stimulation of other cranial nerves induced much weaker electric waves, of much smaller distribution.

The Chinese researchers then experimented by ignoring the acupuncture points and stimulating the areas rich in nerve endings, even the peripheral nerves, with equally satisfactory results. It was further discovered that the closer the stimulus was applied to the site of operation, the better the anaesthetic effect. The results of manual stimulation by twirling the acupuncture needle were compared with electro-acupuncture (using a simple pulse-stimulator connected to the acupuncture needles), and it was found that the anaesthetic effect was almost the same.

The ear and external ear canal, which played such a key part in electro-acupuncture anaesthesia, is a highly innervated area, supplied by sensory fibres of the seventh and tenth cranial nerves. The nerve endings are closely interwoven and superimposed on each other. Since these nerves have a very wide distribution, the investigators put forward the hypothesis that stimulation of the branches in the ear had a reflex effect on practically all parts of the body.

Electrical stimulation in the West

Electrically-induced anaesthesia was not new to the West, nor even introduced by China. Research for an alternative to chemical anaesthesia was begun as early as 1902 in the Hospital Necker in Paris, France, where Professor Francois Leduc discovered that certain high-frequency electric currents had an anaesthetizing effect. By 1966 (when the first International Symposium of Electro-Anaesthesia and Electro-Sleep was held in Europe) Professor Aimé Limoge, on the faculty of dental surgery at the University of Paris, had designed a high-frequency generator that would keep a patient anaesthetized for as long as necessary. Unlike electro-convulsive therapy, where the current is of short duration and the patient remains unconscious for some time afterwards, in electrical anaesthesia the patient could have a long period of current and awake immediately it was stopped.[190]

In England, in 1967, Professors Patrick Wall and W. H. Sweet reported successful treatment of eight patients with severe cutaneous pain by electrical stimulation of their peripheral nerves.[333] The following year W. H. Sweet and J. G. Wespic reported success in 18 patients with intermittent peripheral stimulation[306] (see Appendix II, note 2). Then in 1974 Drs Wall and Nathan described treating 30 patients suffering from post-herpetic neuralgia with prolonged self-administered electric stimulation from a portable apparatus. The results were good in 11 cases. In eight of these the course of the neuralgia was improved, and two were cured.[217] From their studies, Wall and Sweet produced their 'gate theory' of pain control (see Appendix II, note 3).

Twenty years previously scientists in the Soviet Union had developed a new method of 'neurotropic therapy', or electro-sleep. It had been preceded, in the USSR and other countries in Eastern Europe, by numerous physiological studies of the effects of electric current on the animal and human brain.

Sleep therapy, based on Pavlov's concept of sleep as protective inhibition, was widely acclaimed as an important addition to therapeutic measures, comparing favourably with the disadvantages associated with drug-induced sleep. However, in spite of the acceptance of electro-sleep as a therapeutic method both in the USSR and Europe, its widespread success in clinical practice, and extensive theoretical and experimental research (over 450 publications at that time), no uniformity of viewpoint emerged, either on the mechanism of electro-sleep induction or on the mechanism of its therapeutic effect.

I was interested in one example given by a Russian doctor, G. V. Sergeev of the Institute of Internal Medicine, USSR Academy of Medical Sciences, Moscow, in a paper entitled 'The use of electro-sleep in clinical medicine' in which he said 'Electro-sleep, as a factor exerting a neurotropic action on the central nervous system, is used in clinical medicine for the treatment of various diseases with underlying disturbances of the cortical regulation of somatic function.'

He described his electro-sleep technique: '... rectangular pulse, constant polarity, duration of pulse 0.2–0.3 msec, current intensity 15–20 mA expressing the amplitude value of the pulse at a frequency of 80–100 pulses per sec., daily sessions lasting from 30 minutes to 2 hours, course of treatment of up to 20–25 sessions.'

Brain waves and frequencies

Such ongoing investigations by scientists from East and West, as well as the emergence of biofeedback techniques, provided fascinating and tantalizing clues to the mystery of drug addicts being 'cured' by our electro-acupuncture in Hong Kong. But one which stood out above others in my thinking was the work of Dr W. Grey Walter, the noted neurophysiologist.[334] He was the first to correlate the frequencies of the brain's electrical waves with epileptic seizures and to describe the now well-known 'alpha' and other brain rhythms associated with mood changes (see Appendix II, note 4).

That was the connection I needed: between electrical stimulation, brain waves (cycles per second, frequencies, hertz) and the alterations of mood – such as those induced by drugs. If I could find the coordinates of electrical frequencies and brain cycles, in much the same manner as Grey Walter had done with his epileptics, I would solve the mystery (see Appendix II, note 5).

About the same time as Grey Walter in Bristol was making his major advance in the understanding of epilepsy (1950), Dr Irving Cooper in New York was reading a book by the Italian physiologist, Giuseppe Moruzzi, who made the remarkable observation that electrical stimulation of the anterior lobe of the cerebellum could produce either an increase or decrease of decerebrate rigidity from the same point, depending on the frequency of stimulation. He found that with frequencies of 10 Hz, increase of decerebrate rigidity might be activated, while frequencies of 100 to 300 Hz invariably produced a decrease. Also, the decrease of frequency of stimulation could be compensated for by increasing the duration of each stimulus. However a train of repetitive stimulation was always necessary in order to produce an inhibitory or facilitatory effect.

Then 20 years later, in the winter of 1972, Dr Cooper began implanting electrodes on the cerebellum by a surgical technique called suboccipital craniotomy for cases of severe epilepsy and various spastic conditions. It was these operations and findings that we discussed during his visit to Hong Kong in February 1973.

He had concluded that cerebellar stimulation arrested both the clinical seizures and the concomitant ictal EEG discharge, and that this suggested a possible cerebellar interference with electrical seizure discharge, as had already been demonstrated in animal experiments. Such a finding was in keeping with other observations of cerebellar function. For example, anterior cerebellar stimulation did not appear clinically to affect muscular tone in normal limbs, but did lessen tone in spastic extremities (see Appendix II, note 6).

Over a period of two years of such stimulation he found that there were no signs of undesirable motor, sensory, intellectual or emotional changes.[68]

So, from the best of the West and the best of the East, in 1973 I had arrived at a working rationale with which to investigate the possibility of a cure for drug addictions.

Chapter 6
Fitting the jigsaw together

Encounters with drug addiction

To the best of my knowledge I had never seen a drug addict until I reached Hong Kong in 1964. There at the Chinese Tung Wah Hospital, the largest hospital group in Asia, the problems associated with drug addiction became a daily part of my professional life. I have had as many as 11 patients on some form of opiates in a ward of 14 people; admittedly, this was an unusually high ratio, but 10 to 15 patients on narcotics in a larger ward was a regular occurrence. In 1964 the official number of opiate addicts in Hong Kong was admitted to be 100,000 in a population of under 4,000,000. Those with experience of the drug problem said the figure was much higher.

I had come into contact with the drug problem earlier through George who had gone to China as a missionary in 1946, right after World War II. While there, and later during three years of living and travelling in Tibet, he had seen a great deal of drug addiction - mostly opium smoking or the swallowing of opium pills.

After obtaining my Fellowship of the Royal College of Surgeons in Edinburgh, I had gone straight to India. I taught and practised general surgery from 1948 to 1953 at the Christian Medical College in Ludhiana, Punjab. I met George in 1952 during a holiday visit to the Indian-Tibetan border town of Kalimpong in the Himalayas of North Bengal. We were married in September 1953 during a leave in Aberdeen, Scotland.

When we returned to India in 1954 - to Kalimpong where George was based while writing his articles and books, and doing lay preaching in various parts of India with indigenous Indian Christian leaders - I had no hospital in which to practise major surgery adequately. In 1956 I agreed to be superintendent of the Indian Tea Association central hospital in Darjeeling, some 30 miles from Kalimpong, with responsibility for over 100 small outlying tea-garden hospitals. I was there for four years. For my work in building the central unit into a very effective community hospital I received a Member of the British Empire award from Her Majesty, Queen Elizabeth.

George and I returned to England in 1961, partly because I was eight months pregnant with our second child, and partly because George wanted to enter politics. While in London, George was unexpectedly brought into contact with the drug problem again, this time through the late Hephzibah Menuhin, Yehudi's pianist sister, and her sociologist husband, Richard Hauser, both deeply involved with the problems of violence and drug abuse among the youth of London.

In January 1964, George left Britain to film a series of television documentaries in Asia. One of those, 'Raid Into Tibet' was an account of Tibetan guerrilla activities against the Chinese occupation army inside Tibet from bases in the high Himalayas of Nepal. During this period I practised surgery at the United Mission Hospital in Kathmandu, the capital of Nepal.

George and his television colleagues then went on to make a film about 'The Opium Trail' from 'the golden triangle' in northeast Burma and Thailand, to Hong Kong. At that time Hong Kong was said to have the world's worst drug problem. A 300-milligram packet of heroin, containing 40 per cent heroin and 60 per cent barbiturate, cost less than a pack of cigarettes and was as easily obtained. Almost any side alley had its drug vendor, who was prepared either to inject drugs by syringe or to sell them in powder form three times a day - or as often as wanted. The schools and colleges became riddled with drug abuse as dealers peddled their drugs like candy-sellers outside the playgrounds and playing fields.

I was aware of all this through George, who not only continued to amass information - he had been asked to write a definitive book on the drug problem by the Hong Kong government - but who was also in demand to talk to school groups, parents and church youth classes, in addition to his professional talks on radio and television.

Initial trials of the treatment

So when Dr Wen asked George to provide known drug-addicts willing to test electro-acupuncture as a treatment for their addiction, I became involved in these first trials.

Over a period of three months, from January to March, 1973, we treated 40 cases of drug addiction in the Tung Wah Hospital in our spare time. Thirty of these patients were opium addicts, and the others were heroin addicts. Six of these 40 cases came voluntarily for treatment of drug addiction; the remainder were in hospital for a variety of other conditions. The amount of drugs taken varied considerably among individuals. (The official average daily drug intake in Hong Kong was worth HK$8.60 (about £1). At that time this amount would buy 900 milligrams of the heroin-barbiturate mixture – that's over £60 at mid-1980s prices.)

We modified the standard acupuncture techniques of inserting needles in hand, wrist and ears for inducing surgical analgesia by using needles in the patients' ears only. In acupuncture terminology we used the 'lung' point in the middle of the concha, and here we inserted needles in each ear between the skin and the cartilage for a depth of a quarter of an inch, then connected the needles by crocodile clips and leads to the electrical stimulator. The current intensity was increased until the patient felt a slight, not unpleasant tingling in the ear, and this was continued for an average of 30 to 40 minutes per treatment, two or three treatments a day to begin with, given for five days during the acute withdrawal stage, followed by one treatment for the subsequent four or five days.

About 10 to 15 minutes after stimulation began, the patient's watering eyes and running nose became dry; the aching, shivering and abdominal pain decreased; breathing became regular, and the patient began to feel warm and relaxed.

Dr Wen and Dr Cheung reported the results in *The Asian Journal Of Medicine*:

> Of the 40 cases, 39 were discharged and are free of drug addiction. These patients have gained weight and said that they have since had no urge to take the drug. Twenty-two of these cases had their urine sent for investigation to see if it was positive for drugs. The report showed one doubtful case, and one positive case ... The 'doubtful' result related to a case of concussion, who had been put on Luminal for post-concussional syndrome. The only positive case was suffering from tumour of the bladder, which necessitated injections of narcotic to stop his pain. The 20 cases which showed negative urine tests are free of the drug and so far have no urge for it either ... Up to the present, eight cases have come back to have one or two repetitions

> of treatment ... Each of them was given the treatment as an out-patient, and so far they have no recurrence of the symptoms.[330]

Over the next four months we treated more than 100 cases of heroin and opium addiction, with similar results (see Appendix II, note 7).

NEW HOPE FOR ADDICTS

The successful treatment of these patients, together with others I was treating privately in Hong Kong, opened up new hope for possible cures of hitherto intractable conditions. In so many ways, Hong Kong was the ideal place in which to conduct such research, with its fine hospitals and a huge drug problem. Yet the official attitude towards the drug problem was almost paranoid. Because of political, social and financial factors, Hong Kong authorities seemed more concerned with concealing the scale of the problem than with finding a possible medical solution.

Pressure was applied on Dr Wen, Dr Cheung and myself to stop all experiments with acupuncture anaesthesia, but because acupuncture, as a traditional Chinese form of medicine, was allowed by law to be practised in Hong Kong, it could not be stopped legally. Strongly worded circulars issued by official medical authorities threatened us with severe consequences; there were warnings against our giving public lectures (after Dr Wen had given one to a packed audience of doctors). There was also pressure through the hospital (where we were conducting our research in addition to our own surgical responsibilities), and official denials to the local and international press that anything medically significant in the area of drug addiction cure had happened, although several reports had already appeared in the *New York Times* and the London *Observer*.

Our research and the reports in the media had emphasized the use of acupuncture, mainly because of the widespread interest following on James Reston's article, and the subsequent articles by doctors accompanying President Nixon. But I was increasingly convinced from my reading and personal observations that acupuncture was not the key to the success of the treatment. Rather, some unknown electrical factor associated with frequencies was producing the results. From my own Chinese medical colleagues, who knew a great deal about the history and practice of traditional acupuncture, I knew that it was not effective in treating drug addictions, although it did help with muscle relaxation.

From my reading and widening clinical experience I had become increasingly convinced that it was electrical stimulation of nerve pathways, rather than the system of electro-acupuncture, which was the important factor in the addiction curative process. For example, when experimenting with the electrical current by varying the frequencies and wave forms, I found that certain frequencies were dramatically effective while with other patients the same frequencies were woefully inadequate. Chinese addicts given a treatment of 111 Hz on the Chinese model 6.26 stimulator would respond positively, describing the sensation as being like an average shot of heroin. Yet treatment at that frequency had little or no effect on amphetamine addicts.

I resolved, therefore, to design my own machine with a much wider range of frequencies and wave forms, and have it built to my own specifications, which would allow me to experiment. I was now receiving reports of exciting developments from researchers investigating electrical stimulation in other countries, which increased my interest even more.

Research in China

Inside China, the Kuang-si Medical College Group published a report of investigations carried out on 52 normal animals, in the *Scientia Sinica.* The anaesthetic effect of acupuncture was compared before and after the administration of a variety of drugs affecting the nervous system, and it was found that some increased the effectiveness of acupuncture anaesthesia, whereas others invariably reduced it (see Appendix II, note 8).

Another group of Chinese researchers in Peking Medical College filmed a series of experiments with rabbits,[261] which I saw when it was shown in Hong Kong. They studied the parts played by various brain chemicals in acupuncture analgesia, especially the effects of substances that were known to be involved in the transmission of nerve impulses and thus were probably concerned in both pain and analgesia.

The film showed two rabbits with their circulations linked. Only one received acupuncture to induce analgesia, yet the pain threshold was raised significantly in both animals. In another experiment, cerebrospinal fluid from one acupunctured rabbit was transferred to a non-acupunctured rabbit. The pain threshold of the second rabbit was considerably increased, though not as greatly as in the first rabbit.

Acupuncture by finger pressure was used on the rabbits rather than the widely-known needles, since needles caused too much local tissue damage. Some Chinese claim that historically finger acupuncture was probably the first method used, and it was coming back into favour. This film gave me the first indication that needles might not be necessary - that surface electrodes could be used.

Later reports in the West confirmed the importance of these observations. The London *Times* Science Report of 28 March 1974, discussing articles published in the Chinese journal *Scientia Sinica*, declared:

> As well as providing valuable and interesting evidence that the mechanism of acupuncture analgesia is different from that mediated by morphine, the parallel experiments run with morphine show that the methods of investigation and measurement that the authors are pursuing are valid, and that the conclusions they draw are to be considered seriously. There seems little doubt that acupuncture produces changes that result in the blocking of pain impulses in the brain.[281]

Research in the West

Researchers in the West were also finding in their rat and cat experiments that when animals were stimulated through electrodes placed in the periaqueductal grey area, they 'become totally unresponsive to pain while retaining a normal ability to respond to other stimuli and that the effect out-lasted the stimulation by several hours'[205] (see Appendix II, note 9).

I had kept in touch with Dr Cooper by correspondence, and he told me of treating a patient with severe action myoclonus of three years' duration, a sequel of cerebral anoxia. For the first few weeks after implantation and stimulation at 200 Hz there was no improvement, but improvement did come gradually, so that within a few months of continuous stimulation her totally incapacitating generalized twitching had virtually disappeared. He had also treated about 30 other patients suffering from hypertonic states such as cerebral palsy, the consequences of stroke, and various forms of spastic paralysis, as well as intractable epilepsy, all with dramatic success. The technique he used was to implant electrodes in the brain by surgery, and to control stimulation of the cerebellum by what he termed 'the prosthetic mobilization of the inhibitory potential of the cerebellar cortex' (that is, making use of hitherto untapped functions of the cerebellum by means of electrical stimulation).

'The cerebellum is an inhibitory mechanism functioning somewhat as a rheostat,' Dr Cooper explained. 'It has a modulating function on the rest of the brain. The evidence for its function has built up over the years in animal experiments. What is new is the application of some of this knowledge to human disease.'

Dr Cooper devised the 'Cooper Brain Pacemaker' to cure neural disorders. Plates of silicone-coated Dacron mesh, to which were attached four to eight pairs of platinum disc electrodes, were surgically placed on the patients' cerebellar cortex (see Appendix II, note 10). The electrode plates were connected with subcutaneous leads to a small radio-frequency receiver that was implanted in the patient's chest before brain surgery began. Electrode stimulation originated from a transmitter carried outside the body, and occurred by trans-epidermal inductive coupling by means of an antenna taped to the patient's chest directly over the receiver. The transmitter, about the size of a pack of cigarettes, could be carried in a pocket or purse.

Dr Cooper doubted that the natural course of cerebral palsy, or of the other diseases he was treating, would be changed by cerebellar stimulation. However, he did feel that 'prosthetic stimulation of the cerebellum may gradually recondition reflex functioning of some brain circuits'.

He had observed behavioural changes in all his patients, even in the few who had had little or no physical improvement. All of his patients were independently evaluated before and after surgery and in continued follow-up, and exhibited the following behavioural changes:

(1) reduced tension, anxiety and feeling of stress;
(2) improved rationality and fluency of speech;
(3) reduced depression, and increased optimism;
(4) reduced feelings of anger and of aggressive outbursts associated either with seizures or between seizures, and improved emotional control.[68]

A scientific jigsaw puzzle

The many pieces of the scientific jigsaw puzzle portraying electrical stimulation were beginning to fit together. A strong connection had already been made between electrical stimulation and pain, emotion and altered states of consciousness. A connection appeared highly probable between electrical stimulation and drugs of addiction, with their altered emotions and states of consciousness.

I read a series of 'Skinner box' experiments investigating causes of drug dependence in rats. A stimulating electrode was permanently implanted in the medial forebrain bundle of the brain, so that this bundle of neurons was stimulated whenever the rat pressed a lever. This indicated noradrenaline as the main mediator of reward (see Appendix II, note 11). Such experiments supported the theory that drugs of dependence induced euphoria by enhancing production of noradrenaline (and related catecholamines) in the brain. The important question for me was whether electrical stimulation produced the same results in humans.

Dr H. O. J. Collier, a British scientist, described the significance of the 'Skinner box' experiments in drug dependence:

> In animals whose psychic processes are observable through their behaviour we may speak of 'behavioural dependence' which may include psychic and physical components ... An animal is usually prepared in dependence studies with an intravenous cannula connected to an infusion pump, which is activated by a lever in the wall of the cage. By pressing the lever the animal can self-inject drugs ... If the animal is offered a strong instead of a weak solution of heroin the pattern of its lever-pressing will be different. It will learn to press the lever more and more often.
>
> An analogy can be drawn between self-injection of a rewarding drug and the behaviour seen when the animal is prepared so that it can stimulate electrically a certain point in its own brain ... In this situation a rat usually stimulates its brain several times an hour ... In the most general terms, a multiplication induced by the drug of dependence of some kind of receptor or enzyme, carrier, neurone, or storage site that handles, or reacts to, an active endogenous substance mediating or modulating neuronal responses, appears to be nearest to explaining dependence.[64]

In March 1973, Dr Solomon Snyder and researcher Candace Pert of the Johns Hopkins University School of Medicine in Baltimore, reported in *Science* that they had succeeded in locating in the brain the receptor sites that attracted opioids.[245] The area of the brain with the heaviest concentration of opioid receptors was the *corpus striatum*, which seems to play a part in integrating motor activity and perceptual information. The receptors occurred much less frequently in the cerebral cortex, which regulates higher intellectual functions, and in the brain stem, which controls sleeping and wakefulness.

Snyder concluded that the ideal opioid agonist should be potent, long-lasting, non-addictive, orally administered and free from side-effects. When given over a period of time to an ex-addict such a substance would, he hoped, decondition heroin-seeking behaviour and possibly result in psychological changes as well.

I wondered if such a hope might be found, not only in some chemical substance, but in electrical stimulation? From the beginning of experimentation the idea had been implicit that the use of electricity for stimulation could produce physiological activity. There was every reason, therefore, for the idea of stimulation to be introduced in current medical thinking, even though the results of such stimulation differed from normal physiological responses.

A leading article in *The Lancet*, discussing the 'sheer technical trickery' of using an implanted electrode to determine normal functioning in an individual, concluded:

> There seems to be no reason why not. When Delgado, using such stimulation, stopped a charging bull at a gallop, what was arresting was not only the bull's deceleration, but also the fact that the bull's rage was turned off ... It looked as though a physiological effect had been produced on the animal's behaviour. This limbic lobe, which has taken over automatic and emotional or temperamental functions, acts in a simple on-off way over a long time scale, and seems eminently suitable for true stimulation. Although many parts of it have been stimulated, our knowledge of the possibilities of long-term stimulation has hardly begun, despite the fact that Delgado and co-workers have made many investigations on animals including primates, and even a few human beings.[16]

The same *Lancet* leading article described a case of spontaneous pain arising from a 'predominantly cortical' lesion which was relieved by intermittent electrical stimulation through an electrode stereotactically implanted in or near the internal capsule:

> The temporal cortex, as in all reported cases of this sort, was known to be damaged and the patient showed loss of right-parietal activity

> – that is, of functions on the left side of the body. The stimulating electrode was reckoned to be in the posterior limb of the internal capsule. Bipolar stimulation with waves of 0.25 msecs, 100 to 150 per second, 1.5 to 2.5 volts, produced a sensation of light tingling and vibration. After five to fifteen minutes, pain and an unpleasant spreading dysaesthesia disappeared, to remain at bay for one to twenty-six hours. *The exact form of the electrical current is important.* With these characteristics and the symptoms experienced by the patient it is likely that true stimulation was produced. (my italics)

STRUCTURAL CHANGES

Earlier experiments in England by Dr L. S. Illis of Southampton had also demonstrated possible structural changes after electrical stimulation (see Appendix II, note 12). I wrote to him regarding his experiments with electrical stimulation, describing some of my own experience. He replied:

> I was particularly interested in your comments about the possibility of electrical stimulation altering tissue growth. I thought you might be interested in some work showing the effect of repetitive stimulation on the central nervous system. Since publishing that paper I have come across two further reports of similar experiments, with similar results – re a structural change after stimulation.

Dr Robert Becker, Professor of Orthopedic Surgery at the Upstate Medical Center, New York State, and Medical Investigator at the Veterans Administration Hospital, Syracuse, New York, was a leading international authority on electrical stimulation as well as an expert on the subject of tissue regeneration. Having succeeded in stimulating regeneration in laboratory animals, Dr Becker had begun to apply his technique to humans for fractured bones showing non-union.

Becker's work in tissue regeneration dated back to 1958 when he and his colleagues began experiments to determine whether electrical stimulation could trigger bone and other tissue growth in animals. Earlier research had already established that the chances of regeneration in a species depended on the proportion of nerve tissue in the areas of regeneration. Becker pointed out the inability of man, with roughly 70 per cent of his total nerve mass concentrated in his brain, to regenerate, whereas salamanders, with half the mass of their nerve tissue in their brains and the remainder distributed throughout their bodies, can grow new tails, legs, and even heart tissue. Becker put forward the hypothesis that he could increase the regenerative powers of higher animals, somehow compensating for the small proportion of nerve tissue in their extremities, by bolstering the electrical activity in the nerve network. After amputating limbs from 39 rats he planted electrodes in the amputation sites and applied current to stimulate cell changes. All but two of the rats responded with some limb growth; many regenerated amputated forelegs as far as the first joint.[27]

At a symposium on bioelectrochemistry in France, Becker further expanded his hypothesis to postulate 'a complete operational system existing in living organisms which controls such basic functions as growth, healing and biological cycles'. He described the system as 'a data transmission system in an analog fashion using varying levels of direct current as its signal. The system interlocks physically with the nervous system and is postulated to be its precursor.' The direct current system is linked to the nervous system, and to all body cells. 'The concept explains the biological effects of applied electrical currents including: *electrical anaesthesia, electrical growth control and electro-acupuncture*. It also furnishes a testable hypothesis for predicting other effects that might be of clinical significance.'[28] (my italics) (See Appendix II, note 13.)

A difficult decision

Although I now felt that I had enough information for a working hypothesis and a possible rationale for electrical stimulation as a successful treatment for chemical substance addiction, I was in a more difficult situation than either Dr Cooper or Dr Becker. Dr Cooper was a neurosurgeon attached to a training hospital and Dr Becker was an orthopaedic surgeon attached to a research laboratory. Whereas both were well known in the United States, as well as worldwide, I was a general surgeon who had spent the past 25 years doing all kinds of surgery in sometimes primitive conditions in Asia and was unknown in the field of addictions.

But after nine months of treating over 100 Hong Kong addicts by electro-acupuncture with dramatic effect, and reading widely of the growing importance of the electrical stimulation of nerve pathways, I was faced with the difficult choice of either abandoning my surgery, which I loved, or giving up a medical possibility which far exceeded my surgery in importance.

I decided to leave surgery and Hong Kong and return to London to pursue my research into what I was already calling NeuroElectric Therapy, or NET for short. In 1973 I started practising in London's medical mecca - Harley Street.

Chapter 7
Development of NET

My early research in Britain

Most of my time after returning to England in 1973 was devoted to reviewing the material written on electrical stimulation of various kinds in different countries and to developing my own neuro-electric stimulator.

The personal interest and cooperation of several friends and patients enabled me to continue with my research. Violinist Yehudi Menuhin, for example, introduced me to his friend, Andrew Grima, jeweller to the Queen, who worked with me for several months to design a suitable ear-clip incorporating a needle so tiny that it caused no pain. (I had found that my European patients could not tolerate the pain of the Chinese acupuncture needles in their ears.)

Another friend of Yehudi Menuhin, David Shackman of Shackman Instruments Limited, put all his firm's facilities at my disposal. His managing director, Geoff Bennett, patiently worked with me to produce a stimulator built to my specifications. I had tried the only stimulators available in Britain at that time (all imported from the United States) and found them useless for my purposes. But Geoff Bennett knew nothing of biology, naturally, and I knew nothing of electronics.

HISTORICAL ANTECEDENTS

From my reading I had learned that electrophysiology as a term and as a science originated in the sixteenth century. At about the same time that Galileo was inventing the compound telescope and establishing a new cosmology, an English physician, William Gilbert, was combining his practice of medicine with investigations of magnetism and 'electricity' - a word coined by Gilbert. He also invented the first instrument for measuring electric fields, the electroscope.

The eighteenth century brought an upsurge of interest in electricity, and Stephen Hales, one of several clergymen with an interest in science, suggested that nerves functioned by conducting 'electrical powers'. The Abbé Nolet tried to cure paralysis by electricity, and Abraham Bennet invented a 'gold-leaf electroscope' for detecting and measuring electric charges.

In 1775, Luigi Galvani in Italy began his experiments in electricity and biology, and the first of a series of extraordinary 'accidents' occurred. In 1786 one of Galvani's assistants, while dissecting a frog's legs, happened to touch the nerve to the muscles with his scalpel while a static electrical machine was operating on a table nearby. This made the muscle contract, thereby launching a period of major advances in the understanding of electricity and biology. Before the end of the century Galvani's nephew, Giovanni Aldini, a physicist, reported treating a patient suffering from a personality disorder by administering currents to the head. The patient's personality steadily improved and eventually he was completely healed.

In Copenhagen, Denmark, Hans Christian Oersted noticed, while giving a lecture, that every time he produced an electrical current the needle of a demonstration compass lying on the table moved. From that chance observation he developed a series of experiments to demonstrate electromagnetism.

In the nineteenth century Carlo Matteucci, an Italian professor of physics, proved beyond doubt that an electrical current was generated by injured tissues. An experimenter in Berlin working for Johannes Müller, the world's foremost physiologist at that time, duplicated Matteucci's experiment, and went beyond it. He discovered that when a nerve was stimulated, a measurable electrical impulse was produced at the site of stimulation and travelled at high speed down the nerve, causing the muscle to contract.

In the twentieth century, the interest of two American doctors already mentioned, Cooper and Becker, in the work of Matteucci and other Italian scientists led to the development of their work in cerebellar and bone electrical stimulation.

As in earlier centuries, 'accidental' discoveries played a role in the advance of scientific knowledge. Cooper, described as 'the father of cryogenic surgery', conceived of that technique while opening a bottle of wine with a carbon dioxide bottle opener. In 1967, Becker described how, while studying the electrical factors associated with fracture healing, 'a regenerative-type growth process in the frog was inadvertently discovered by our group'[29]. And of course our discovery that electro-acupuncture 'cured' addictions was made while we were experimenting with analgesia, an entirely different field.

BIOELECTRIC TREATMENTS TODAY

Now electrical stimulation is also applied in a wide variety of treatment processes, sometimes in very complicated forms. It has been established that the administration of electrical current in small amounts which are only mildly stimulating has beneficial effects in:

- epilepsy and spasticity (with electrodes implanted on the cerebellar cortex)[67];
- non-union of bone fractures (with electrodes implanted in the bone adjacent to the fracture site)[28, 108];
- intractable skin ulcers (with electrodes applied to the ulcer)[163, 275];
- general anaesthesia (with electrodes above the bridge of the nose and behind the ears)[49];
- control of chronic pain (with electrodes applied locally in the area of pain, or segmentally)[103, 194, 211];
- urinary incontinence (with electrodes inserted as a needle into the perineum or in an anal plug)[114];
- to rehabilitate paralysed muscles, and the bladder in particular, in multiple sclerosis (with percutaneous electrodes in the epidural space[66, 151] or externally over the lower spine);
- to relieve spasticity and clonus in amyotrophic lateral sclerosis (by electrical subcutaneous nerve stimulation)[332];
- to accelerate union of divided nerves and perhaps the spinal cord (using electromagnetic fields - EMF)[27, 175, 256, 345];
- to cause skin vasodilation in peripheral ischaemia such as Raynaud's disease and diabetic polyneuropathy (with electrodes applied to the affected limb)[164];
- malignant lung tumours (with needle electrodes inserted into tumour)[224];
- I and others also use it for muscle and joint injuries and local infections.

I have just noticed in today's *Times* as I write this that the Queen has been treated with a pulsed EMF machine for a strained shoulder and 'was cured with two 90-minute sessions'[314].

My own research continues

During the years 1973 to 1975 Geoff Bennett and I developed two machines which gave me an increasing number of accurate responses based on my working hypothesis, but it was very hit or miss. It was more hit than miss, however, with enough hits to convince me that my hypotheses and researches in the exciting new field of bioengineering were a possible major step toward a cure for the scourge of addictions.

The second 'Shackman–Patterson' machine which we developed had a variety of wave-forms, pulse widths from 0.1 to 1.5 msecs, and frequencies varying from 5 to 2,000 Hz. This transistorized machine included both the standard square or rectangular wave-form used in most bio-electric treatments and in intracranial implantations, and the spike form used by the Chinese. They, presumably - although it is not stated in any publication available outside China - had some special reason for using this particular form. Although empirically I found the rectangular wave-form more effective, I still consider the precise shape of wave important; some laboratory researchers have produced an effect with triangular pulses that was unobtainable with rectangular pulses.[168] Our machine could also insert a modulation of 50 KHz (I discovered later that French researchers were inserting a 100 KHz modulated signal in their electro-anaesthesia machine[239]).

In the first six months of research, from November 1973 to June 1974, I concluded that twirling of the acupuncture needle produced a mild electrical current, thereby altering the electrical phenomena occurring in every nerve cell. Clinical evidence indicated that NET might be producing regeneration of neurons, or, at least, a reconditioning of some brain circuits, such as the reticular formation.

I discussed those ideas with Professor Patrick Wall, one of the formulators of the 'gate theory' of pain. He was reluctant to accept the possibility that I could be regenerating brain tissue. Yet, he said, it seemed clear that I was affecting the brain circuits in some specific way. In my opinion, this could only be due to some chemical being released by brain cells because of the constant delay of 10 to 15 minutes before an addict starting NET experienced any relief of withdrawal symptoms.

In Hong Kong in 1972–3 when we had treated heroin and opium addicts who were showing acute withdrawal symptoms, we noticed that the signs of withdrawal began to diminish about 10–15 minutes after beginning treatment. In another five or ten minutes some patients even fell asleep. In a total of 30 minutes or so all were comfortable and happy. We therefore set 30 minutes as a recommended time for any one treatment; but in London, I increased that to a basic 40 minutes for outpatient treatment.

I encouraged inpatients, both alcohol and drug addicts, to keep the machine on continuously if possible. By the time I had developed my third stimulator model, I found that 10 days was enough to treat almost all patients on any drug of addiction, no matter how long they had used the drug, nor how large the daily dosage. Occasionally the 10 days had to be extended when there were complications, either because of the condition of the patient or because of the drug combinations used.

Moreover, the patients I was treating were also undergoing psychological changes for the better. For convenience, I referred to that hypothetical substance as 'Chemical X'. Although I did not know the nature of 'Chemical X', I was encouraged by the continued success in my clinical experience with patients and their rapid and consistent response to the electrical stimulation. After all, most effective medical treatments had emerged in this way, accidentally, and without prior scientific validation. Penicillin was saving lives long before biologists unravelled the precise molecular secrets of how bacteria caused disease. *The Lancet*, discussing the place of intuition and imagination in scientific advances, has stated: 'Many discoveries fundamental to modern science have been the result of a mental flash. Meanwhile, science is retrospective; it proves the educated guess.'

Chemical Breakthrough

In 1975 - one month after the first 'interim report' of my work was published in Europe - another scientific breakthrough was announced, which has since been acclaimed as one of the great discoveries of the century. In Aberdeen University, Scotland, Professor Hans Kosterlitz and Dr John Hughes discovered the presence of a natural substance, enkephalin, in the medial brainstem of rats.[145]

Almost simultaneously their findings were confirmed in Sweden and in the United States by other researchers. Following the discovery of enkephalin, several other naturally occurring substances were discovered and identified and given the generic name of 'endorphins' (from 'endogenous morphine'). The endorphins were substances normally present in the body that acted like morphine. One of them, β-endorphin was demonstrated by Smyth in the Institute of Neurology, London, to be up to 200 times more potent in pain-killing effect than morphine.[291]

Research papers on the endorphins began to appear in a variety of scientific journals as other scientists expanded this major field of investigation. β-endorphin belonged to a class of neuropeptides, many of which are found in areas of the brain known to be involved in the physiology of pain and emotions, and may even be related to some biochemical mechanism involved in mental illness through alterations in the homoeostatic regulation of the naturally occurring substances.[34]

Addiction to opioid drugs like morphine and heroin was assumed by Kosterlitz and Hughes to be the result of some interaction between the natural and synthetic opioid pain-killers. The opioid abstinence syndrome (commonly known as 'withdrawal') can be precipitated within a few minutes by an injection of the drug naloxone. This finding has continued to be a useful tool in identifying endorphin activity in research procedures. These endogenous substances were thought to act as neurotransmitters or neuromodulators at synaptic junctions of neurons, but unlike morphine they are very rapidly destroyed in the brain by enzymes.[176]

One of the unsatisfactory features of prolonged administration of the endorphins, natural or synthetic, is that they induce tolerance and dependency just as other opioids do, and cross-tolerance develops between morphine and endorphins. This has diminished earlier hopes that the discovery of endorphins would lead to the synthesis of pain-killing drugs that would produce neither tolerance nor dependency.

On the other hand, the discovery of endorphins increased the potential of my NeuroElectric stimulation immensely. Dr Kosterlitz had been my tutor at Aberdeen University so I arranged to meet him to talk about my own research findings. He was tremendously interested and made a number of helpful suggestions. He also told me of other scientists who were working with electrical stimulation and enkephalin, and agreed that my 'Chemical X' was possibly enkephalin.

My theory was that by competing for the opioid receptors in the brain, synthetic opioids led to a gradual decrease in production of the natural enkephalins. Hence, a person using opioids regularly needed an increasing dose of synthetic opioids to make good the loss, creating the condition of tolerance. This diminishing of the body's natural opioids and the consequent need to ingest more synthetic opioids created the typical 'drug hunger' of the addict, and the 'craving' or withdrawal symptoms when the synthetic drug was withheld.

According to Kosterlitz and Hughes, a consistently maintained dosage of morphine stopped the release of enkephalin from the neurons through some feedback mechanism. This new theory concerning the mechanism of the addiction process explained the brain's dependency on morphine as a substitute for its own naturally occurring painkiller, enkephalin.[144]

I could now see a possible link between Kosterlitz and Hughes' feedback mechanism, Becker's 'hybrid data transmission and control system', and Melzack's 'central biasing mechanism', influencing transmission at all synapses[210] (see Chapter 6, pages 119–20).

Electrical stimulation in animals and humans

Concurrent research into stimulation-produced analgesia (SPA) achieved by implanting electrodes in the brains of animals or humans, and its relationship to the effects on neurotransmitters, elucidated some of my clinical observations in patients undergoing NeuroElectric Therapy (NET), as my own treatment was now called. I had noted that when certain drugs, including narcotics and cocaine, were ingested or injected during a course of NET, the anticipated physical and psychic effects of these drugs were diminished, and occasionally a patient would even experience a very severe aversive effect.

The literature revealed that very powerful analgesia could be produced in rats[111], cats[188] and monkeys[122] by electrical stimulation of certain areas of the brain, particularly the periaqueductal grey area.[187] Significantly, although such stimulation made an animal totally unresponsive to pain, it retained a normal ability to respond to other stimuli.[207] That contrasted with the effects of drugs used clinically for analgesia or narcosis.[205] Nor did stimulation reduce alertness or elicit seizures.[5, 188] Further, it was stimulation and not destruction of the cells which produced the analgesia; actual electrolytic lesions produced different and harmful effects[189, 207, 225] (see Appendix II, note 14).

Dr J.C. Liebeskind, of the University of California, well-known for his work in electrical stimulation, declared the importance of the hypotheses, supported by a considerable amount of evidence, that 'electrical stimulation releases enkephalin or in some other way makes it available for binding at opiate receptor sites, whereas morphine, by resembling the natural substance, interacts with these receptors directly'[187].

Another interesting development in the investigations of the interactions between stimulation-produced analgesia and enkephalin was that the antagonist naloxone reversed the effects of both[145, 146], though not completely in the case of SPA.[6] This was demonstrated in a man whose severe pain was completely controlled through a stereotactically implanted electrode, but who developed acute pain when naloxone was injected and none when a placebo (saline) was injected.[3] The effect was unlikely to have been induced by suggestion, because hypnosis-induced analgesia is not modified by naloxone.[120] Thus, electrical stimulation could obviously control pain without the undesirable effects of drugs usually used for pain.

Excitement in scientific circles ran high over such results. But some researchers felt a need to dampen popular hopes for an immediate cure for addictions, arguing that there was no hope of developing an analgesic peptide with a lessened risk of dependence liability. They saw hope only in developing drugs 'that act indirectly either to activate the enkephalin system or to cause the direct release of enkephalin'[144].

That was exactly what I seemed to be doing with electrical stimulation. Since NET apparently carried with it no dependence liability, I was more hopeful of a possible cure for addiction than many of my more cautious colleagues. Further, to implant electrodes in the brains of drug dependants, or even hardened drug addicts, for stimulation purposes seemed to me to be an unwarranted physical interference. I was already using external stimulation to do the same thing more effectively.

What I now had to find was the most effective external means of delivering the appropriate electrical stimulus to trigger the release of enkephalin. Fifteen months of clinical observations convinced me that the ear-clip I had designed with the tiny needle was as unnecessary as acupuncture needles.[236] Because the electrical stimulus could be transmitted adequately through the skin without needles, I designed a blunt electrode on an ear-clip to be applied to the same area of the concha of the ear. This had the added advantages of eliminating the pain of needling and the risks of local infection or hepatitis transmitted through unsterile needles.[9]

In animals, external electrical stimulation was as effective in altering the activity of opioid receptors as direct stimulation seemed to be.[219] One researcher estimated that 45 per cent of the current applied externally in electro-sleep (where the electrodes were applied fronto-occipital, or fronto-mastoid) passed through the brain, and that an applied current of only one milliampere was sufficient to modify spontaneous firing of neurons.[94] However, Becker and I thought that 45 per cent was an over-estimation, and that 1 per cent was a more reasonable figure.

So the discovery of enkephalin was only the beginning of a whole new branch of science. The finding that the body has receptors to which its own natural opioids attach led to the idea that the body has other receptors to which other chemical substances attach, opening up a whole new world of natural substances, systems and effects.

Indeed, within the next few years, receptors were to be demonstrated for the benzodiazepines (the group of tranquillizers such as Valium and Ativan)[38] and also for the hallucinogens PCP (phencyclidine or 'angel dust') and LSD (d-lysergic acid diethylamide),[10] and an endogenous ligand, or natural substance, for PCP has recently been isolated![255]

That initial idea was a further stimulus to me. I was finding in treating patients that for each group of the different substances of addiction - opioids, alcohol, nicotine, barbiturates, cocaine, marijuana, amphetamines, tranquillizers - a specific electrical frequency was needed to treat that particular addiction.

Uncovering the precise electrical factors for each group of psychoactive drugs, as well as for related conditions such as stress, anxiety, depression and insomnia, demanded extensive laboratory research as well as clinical experience.

Those addicted to narcotics because of severe chronic pain presented yet another problem to be solved. There was no point in detoxifying them from their pain-killers unless NET could also relieve or reduce their pain.

My earlier stimulators

My 'Shackman-Patterson' NeuroElectric stimulator[237] incorporated the most important factors in treating substance addictions:

(1) greater varieties in wave-forms (e.g. in insomnia);

(2) a range of pulse-widths (e.g. in pain control);

(3) frequencies to match different types of drugs (e.g. the stimulant amphetamine group or the depressant opioid group), or the more difficult combination of drugs (e.g. heroin and cocaine), or psychologically associated conditions such as depression and anxiety.

From the surprisingly extensive literature on bioelectricity, I decided that the useful range of frequencies lay within the 1 Hz to 2,000 Hz range which is well clear of the diathermy range beginning at 5,000 Hz or higher. The optimum pulse widths appeared to be between 0.1 and 1.5 milliseconds.

Also, alternating current (AC) seemed preferable to direct current (DC) in order to avoid ionization of tissues, although DC is used in some types of therapy. The use of AC current with no DC bias may be part of the explanation why NET does not cause burns to the skin under the electrodes.

The hoop-shaped blunt electrodes of stainless steel I used in the early stages (conducting area 2.5 millimeters in diameter) were attached to the ear by the clip's tension, with electrode jelly applied to improve conduction. They were held in place by a headset worn either on top of the head, or around the neck, whichever was more comfortable. Patients experienced only a slight and not unpleasant tingling sensation on the skin.

The only adverse side-effect observed in the early years of testing were occasional agitation at the higher frequencies, or, on a few occasions, nausea and headache. But these symptoms were easily reversed by further treatment at a lower frequency, and a reduced current intensity. There were also some unexpected beneficial side-effects. For some reason still not clear to me, the polarity of the current was significant; the patients who claimed better results when the polarity was reversed were all, interestingly, left-handed.

Although I am still puzzled by the importance of polarity in NET (which uses AC with no DC bias), its effects in treatment of other conditions are clear. In infected skin ulcers, when the negative electrode is applied to the ulcer, both infection and healing are suppressed; when the positive (or indifferent) electrode is applied, both are enhanced. The negative is therefore applied to ulcers for the first few days till infection is minimal, and then the positive until healing is complete.[275]

Other examples are for non-union of bone fractures when the negative electrode is implanted at the fracture site and the indifferent electrode applied to adjacent skin.[29] However for malignant lung tumours, the positive is inserted to the centre of the tumour, and the negative to the periphery,[224] thus decreasing cell growth instead of increasing it. Again, nerve growth is enhanced by cathode but unaffected by anode stimulation.[250] In treating pain, the negative electrode is usually applied to the site of pain.

The optimum level of current for addictions has yet to be determined; rat experiments have indicated that high voltage promotes the release of more met-enkephalin than leu-enkephalin on to opioid receptors, whereas low voltage stimulation releases more leu-enkephalin than met-enkephalin.[326]

NO DRUG SUBSTITUTION

From the start of NET treatment I gave no drugs of any kind, and *I cannot overemphasize the importance of this part of the technique.* The drugs of addiction were completely discontinued and no replacement methadone, tranquillizers or sedatives were given. For any patient who had also been using barbiturates I withdrew the barbiturates gradually, because at that time I had not established which frequencies could be relied on to prevent withdrawal convulsions. However, two heavily addicted patients stopped all their barbiturates without reporting it to me, and yet had no convulsions. Both had previously experienced severe withdrawal convulsions when unable to obtain their usual dose of barbiturates.

Later, in 1980 when we had our own clinic and fully trained staff with the knowledge and facilities to treat convulsions should they occur, I stopped all barbiturates and tranquillizers totally and immediately on admission, and gave no anticonvulsant drugs. This new technique was a marked improvement. Only a very few had convulsions, despite having used huge amounts of their drug; in every case, the convulsion lasted only a few seconds, and not one person had a second fit.

It was in Hong Kong that we had the first clinical indication of the mood-altering qualities of varying frequencies. When we changed the frequency from 111 Hz to 250 Hz the Chinese addicts almost immediately reported a sensation of euphoria. The next such observation was in London when an outpatient addict came off his methadone easily after four two-hour sessions, but his addiction to intravenous Ritalin (methylphenidate hydrochloride, an amphetamine-like drug) was undiminished. I had just received the prototype of my first stimulator with a higher range of frequencies, and the first treatment I gave to this patient at 2,000 Hz (a frequency chosen as an educated guess) totally relieved his craving for Ritalin for 18 hours.

When I began using electrical stimulation, I considered that the effect of stopping withdrawal symptoms could be explained by NET's action on the autonomic nervous system, mediated through the vagus nerve which has sensory connections with the external ear canal, the cranial surface of the auricle, and the skin in the region of the mastoid bone. However, this theory of direct parasympathetic modulation did not explain the relief of central signs and symptoms such as restlessness, irritability, muscle aches, yawning and insomnia.[106] Nor did it account for the later results of NET such as the abolition of craving for the drug of addiction after repeated short-term treatments, the increased optimism (in contrast to the usually depressed state of addicts treated by any other method), the freedom from dependence on any other therapeutically used drug, and the rapid and marked improvement in the patient's sleeping pattern without the use of any sedative drugs.

A GOOD NIGHT'S SLEEP

There seemed to be some association with electro-therapeutic sleep, or cerebral electrotherapy (CET), on which considerable research had been done in the Soviet Union and Europe in the previous 20 years. The current in both NET and CET was passed through the brain, though in CET the electrodes were applied so that the current passed through the brain from the forehead region backwards,[25, 294] instead of from side to side as in NET. CET has also been shown to be effective in cases of chronic anxiety, depression and insomnia.[221, 270, 271, 272] Studies had been done with a control series,[277] or a double-blind control series, of patients suffering from neurotic anxiety and depression.[269]

An almost intractable problem in treating substance addictions is the insomnia that follows withholding of the drugs. Natural body rhythms have been so disturbed by drug and life-style abuse that normal patterns of sleep are non-existent. Addicts dread not only the restless nights, but also the intense craving for drugs, and physical agony when they wake up after sleeping fitfully.

Drug addicts claim that it takes about two months to regain a normal sleep pattern after coming off heroin. This has been confirmed physiologically in volunteers who made themselves heroin-dependent.[185] Even though heroin was given to the volunteers for only seven consecutive nights, abnormalities of brain function were detectable for two months after withdrawal. The same study found that morphine suppressed REM sleep,[172] and there was a delayed REM sleep rebound on withdrawal. Some researchers claimed that it might take several months for various bodily functions to return to normal after withdrawal from opioids.[130, 220]

Likewise, after withdrawal from amphetamines, sleep abnormalities take up to two months to disappear,[230] and after barbiturate withdrawal up to four months.[166] Daytime anxieties are reflected in nightmares during sleep. Research studies showed that after only a short period of using a small dose of nitrazepam for insomnia (Mogadon, 5 milligrams), the sleep pattern became more abnormal than it had been before the drug was begun, and reverted to its previous pattern only after one or two weeks.[2, 167]

In 1975, I developed new skin electrodes, similar to those used in ECG applications, and fixed their adhesive surface on the mastoid bone behind the ears. In this way, my NET patients could be given electrical stimulation continuously day and night for the first six days. When patients slept with these electrodes attached, NET effects came more rapidly, sleeping was restful and dreamless, and early morning discomfort was much reduced. Some patients said the NET did not put them to sleep, but that once they were asleep their sleep was deep and free from nightmares. I concluded that some synchronization was occurring between the brain's sleep rhythms and the therapeutic frequency. With these improved techniques most addicts were able to achieve deep restful sleep by the third to the ninth night after commencing NET.[241]

IMPORTANCE OF FREQUENCIES

The importance of frequency was cogently expressed by one well-known scientist: 'The language of the brain is frequency. Some of the implications of this statement are beginning to be understood. Some observations we do not yet understand. When we learn to speak the frequency language of the brain we may begin to understand what it is saying.'[301] Researchers in other applications of medical electronics were coming to similar conclusions[279] (see Appendix II, note 15).

My clinical experience with NET convinced me that the current frequency was the most important factor in treating addictions.

Eric Clapton's willingness to talk about his heroin addiction, and his cure by NET, in 1974, led to dramatic developments. First, two international record companies, the Robert Stigwood Organization and Atlantic Records, began to fund my research; and second, other rock musicians began to come to me for treatment.

The funding was very important to keep the research going, but I also gained vitally important technical information from my rock musician patients. Many of them were experts in acoustic music, electronic synthesizers and the effects of amplification, which meant that they knew a great deal about frequencies and their effects on people's minds and moods.

They were also fascinated to think that their knowledge, combined with mine, could help them free themselves and others from their addictions, so they spent hours experimenting with my NET machine at different frequencies of their own choosing to test and prove the effects on themselves. They confirmed my own impressions that to obtain optimum effects, the pulse frequency had to be changed several times a day, presumably in order to respond to physiological and psychological changes in the course of the treatment.

One musician had used LSD while he was performing before an audience of 52,000 in the United States. He noticed that he could affect himself subjectively and his audience objectively by changing the types of music he played. When he played music with a certain rhythm and tempo he subjectively experienced the audience in colours of black and yellow and red, like a flaming fire; when he changed the music and tempo, he 'saw' the audience as white and blue and felt serenely calm. The audience reacted correspondingly. He had analysed the types of music which produced those effects, and was convinced that it was the frequencies which were significant.

Whenever we hit the right frequencies to 'match' whatever drugs they were addicted to, the musicians would say, 'it just feels right'. If the frequency they chose differed from my choice of frequency, invariably theirs had the best and most immediate effect. Later, this was to be dramatically confirmed in my laboratory work with rats.[46, 47]

I tried the same method for my own very severe and frequent migraine headaches, going through the whole range of frequencies until I found one that felt 'right'. This reduced my migraines to negligible mildness and infrequent occurrence. In treating my migraines I also discovered that the pain eased most when I turned up the voltage sufficiently to cause my occipital muscles to go into clonic spasm - not, by the way, a painful procedure. One hashish addict, in her second treatment, turned up the voltage until most of her scalp muscles were contracting strongly. Afterwards, she told me she felt as if her 'brain had been cleansed'. The parameters of my stimulator were such that there was no danger with this form of experimentation.

Advances in treatment and technology

Towards the end of the 1970s a number of developments changed the course of my research.

The Shackman company, which had been so helpful, felt that my increasingly complex requirements were beyond their production capabilities and suggested that I try to find more expert help elsewhere. Many models of TENS (transcutaneous electrical nerve stimulation) stimulators were by this time available on the USA market. However, these units were for treatment of chronic pain only, and were not only completely inadequate for use in drug withdrawal but also dangerous for application to the head because of the high amount of current they provided. They should be used only on the body or limbs.

A friend introduced me to Peter Loose, whose company was doing more advanced work in electrical technology. Although the company had no experience in what I was doing, Peter was interested and willing to help. I explained the increasingly complex electronic mechanism I now required to effect the desired responses in the patients; this involved combinations and permutations which I had never imagined in my early days of research. So began almost two years' research and experimentation to produce a smaller but more sophisticated and accurate machine than the 'Shackman-Patterson' models. I called them the 'Pharmakon-Patterson Neuro-Electric Stimulator', Models III and IV. The development of these machines continued until early 1980.

Over the years I had tried several times to find funding for a double-blind study of NET, or a control group, to satisfy the usual medical and scientific requirements for any new form of treatment. Although I was not convinced of the usefulness of the double-blind process in this field, I made application to several funding bodies for money to conduct a double-blind trial of NET. Those attempts included applications to the British Medical Research Council and to the National Institute on Drug Abuse in USA. The Medical Research Council were interested and sympathetic but refused my application. (A highly-placed friend told me later that the psychiatrists on the committee had strongly objected to my application on the grounds that I was a surgeon, not a psychiatrist, and hence inadequately prepared to pursue research into the treatment of addictions.) However, the Council officially encouraged me to pursue my investigations in my 'spare time'.

One of the stated reasons for NIDA's refusal was that I had no previous experience of research. Yet I knew of *no* experienced researcher who had a knowledge of NET! The fact is that very few controlled studies have been done to establish the efficacy of any treatment in the drug abuse field. Griffith Edwards, a well-known British psychiatrist in that field (who had appeared in the first BBC film about NET as an independent commentator in 1975), made a proposal for such studies:

> To date in this country, only one major controlled trial has been mounted on an aspect of drug treatment (Mitcheson and Hartnoll, 1978[214]). The most feasible and promising approach might indeed be to mount a series of relatively small scale studies which sequentially assess the effectiveness of particular elements within the total treatment package, either by means of controlled comparison groups *or with patients used as their own controls*.[97] (my italics)

Other experts in the substance abuse treatment field have defended their own and others' failure to do such trials. In a detailed analysis of the USA government-supported Drug Abuse Reporting Program (DARP), analysing 1,496 addicts participating in the research, D. D. Simpson commented:

> Although critics of field research to evaluate treatment outcomes suggest that the use of experimental procedures and randomized control groups is the ideal approach to a scientific determination that a treatment effect does or does not exist, this has not been proved feasible or an acceptable methodological alternative in most research on the effectiveness of drug-abuse treatment.[285]

In my own search of the literature I had found only one controlled study and it was not a double-blind trial. That study used active or simulated cerebral electrotherapy (CET, which I have just described, has a different electronic form and electrode placement from NET) or methadone detoxification, on 28 methadone addicts.

It was reported that 10 of the 13 patients receiving active CET were drug-free by the end of eight to ten days, and that all 13 experienced a marked reduction of their symptoms. The control group did not show significant changes.[121] In addition, double-blind studies of human β-endorphin administered intravenously to addicts undergoing withdrawal from methadone and heroin indicated a reversal of symptoms after the injection and a feeling of normality.[52, 302]

Our first clinic

The second BBC film, 'Still Off The Hook' (see pages 82-3) had been televised in July 1977. It included an interview with the American doctor Richard Corbett eulogizing NET and mentioning that I was being invited to the United States. The broadcast of that film had a dramatic effect. It produced a media outcry against my leaving Britain and taking NET to the United States.

Three offers of funding for research materialized from the showing of this film, the most important of which was from the Rank Foundation. This foundation offered to provide premises and finance for one year's clinical trial in a unit which would reflect my fundamental theories regarding both detoxification[240] and rehabilitation.[238]

It took almost two years to set up a clinic, train an appropriate staff, and prepare the paperwork for future analyses in a treatment process which was so totally new. I devoted myself to preparing the medical instruction and analytical material, while my husband, George, prepared the material for the psycho-spiritual rehabilitation which would complement the rapid detoxification by NET.

During this period, I also met with the late Director of the Marie Curie Memorial Foundation, Dr Don Williams, to discuss possibilities for doing research work on animal models at their Sussex laboratories, investigating the effects of NET in cancer-linked conditions, such as stress and cigarette and alcohol abuse.

The one-year clinical trial took place in 1980, January to December, at a medically-approved, non-profit clinic, Broadhurst Manor in Sussex. The staff was qualified in all respects, and several of the nurses had psychiatric training, but no psychiatrists were employed. The counsellors were chosen on the basis of holding and practising spiritual values in appropriate life situations, and were addressed regularly by my husband out of his own experience of spiritual values analysed and practised in over 40 years in different countries with a variety of religions, customs and ideologies.

There was no pre-selection process for admission for treatment, except for the usual initial medical consultations to establish that the patient had no psychosis or other condition impossible to treat at the clinic.

Having a single unit for detoxification and rehabilitation dramatically increased the benefits of NET, as incoming patients saw others, whom they knew from their own experience should have been suffering, without the usual distress. It quickly became apparent that a whole new national and international approach to the treatment of addictions was going to be necessary because of the rapid detoxification and the subsequent - even concomitant - psychological benefit.

In 1979, while on a visiting professorship to the University of Pennsylvania, I was requested to carry out a short pilot programme at a Government Intermediate Treatment Center in the USA. Half the center was for long-term rehabilitation (12 to 18 months); in the other half of the building, addicts were gradually taken off their drugs with the aid of decreasing doses of methadone. My NET patients, of course, received no drugs at all. At a staff meeting, the Director of Counselling (himself an ex-drug addict and the best counsellor I had come across in any such rehabilitation centre) said:

> I have been questioning your NET patients every day, and I can't believe it - they are sleeping well already! When our addicts are completely drug-free and transferred to the rehabilitation unit, it takes about 2 months before we can do anything with them, they feel so miserable. If we change our method of detoxification to NET, we'll have to change our entire rehab programme to cope with people who are already fit and clear-headed.

The clinical trial I designed for the Pharmakon Clinic, on the basis of my own experience, was actually along the lines which, three years later, Dr Griffith Edwards proposed as ideal (see page 137).

Our move to the United States

When the trial ended in December 1980, we were unable to persuade the British government to integrate the clinic or treatment process within the British system – although in private they were highly complimentary. I decided that my next priority was to produce a statistical analysis of the year's clinical trial, and to begin follow-up research of patients I had treated in the previous seven years in England. Also, George, my husband, had been devising a new and more practical national and international approach to the addiction problem.

One of the biggest obstacles I had found to further development of NET was the negative attitude of people towards any treatment for addictions. From the government (which was having a difficult time finding money for reputable hospitals, and other important medical institutions), to charities (which felt that diseases such as cancer, or organizations for the physically or mentally handicapped should come first), to individuals (who said that addicts deserved to suffer for their self-imposed condition), it was obvious that fund-raising on the scale necessary for research, development, and treatment was not going to be forthcoming in Britain.

Once again an individual with an interest in my work, this time an American, tried to help, and wrote suggesting that we go to America where finance and advanced technology were more available. He was a friend of many years whom my husband had known professionally as a man with worldwide financial and business interests. Now a retired financial adviser, company chairman, inventor, and engineer, he had offered to help us whenever the clinical trial ended.

We went to California in the spring of 1981 where for a number of reasons, including USA patent law, I decided that I would have to design another model of stimulator. For the next few months I worked with Walter Underhill, an electronics engineer, to devise a stimulator which would incorporate a number of new features developed from my years of clinical experience. In addition to his electronics expertise, Walter was able, intuitively and skilfully, to comprehend and solve the problems of turning my increasingly complex theories regarding bioelectric stimulation into technological realities. The new model would be based on my 10 years experience of 'fine-tuning' the stimulator to adapt to the daily, often hourly, changes in response to NET. The complexity of the problem can be judged by the multiplicity of the withdrawal symptoms of each different group of psychoactive drugs (see Appendix III).

My new Model VII NeuroElectric stimulator is not only much more advanced electronically than my previous models, but it also eliminates the principal hindrance to the rapid spread of NET – the necessity for in-depth training of medical personnel. Because it is fully programmed and automated, medical staff – or paramedics, under medical supervision – are now able to use NET effectively, after a careful study of the instruction booklet.

Overall medical supervision is still required because necessary precautions must be taken in the case of patients with heart disease, for example, or in taking patients off drugs which have the potential for causing convulsions in the withdrawal period. There is clinical evidence that NET markedly reduces the incidence of withdrawal convulsions (see Chapter 8, page 156), but my aim in research is to be able to eliminate these completely.

By the end of 1982 I had found funds to complete the statistical analysis of NET addiction treatment over seven years in England; some of the detailed findings were published in the *Journal of Bioelectricity* in May 1984.[242]

While the Pharmakon Clinic trial was going ahead in 1980, I was also deeply involved in the research at the Marie Curie Memorial Foundation Research Laboratories, investigating the biochemical basis of NET. This had been made possible by further financial aid from the rock music world, this time from Pete Townshend and The Who, (which had a reputation for being 'the greatest rock-and-roll group in the world').

Pete had come regularly to visit Eric Clapton while I was treating him and had been so impressed with what NET had done for Eric that he had volunteered to help in any way possible. He and the other members of The Who conducted a series of concerts and donated a large part of the proceeds towards my research. Without all this support the research and results of the trial in the next chapter would never have been completed.

Chapter 8
Research and Results

In the first investigations at the Marie Curie laboratories, NET's dramatic effect in ameliorating restraint stress in rats had been observed. Plasma levels of the adrenal hormone cortisol, which is an indicator of stress, were significantly lower in the NET-treated rats than in the control animals.[48]

Since stress is considered to play a part in the onset of cancer, the optimistic results of NET were of great interest to the Marie Curie researchers, and they extended their investigations into other areas.

Current frequencies

Our research over a four-year period had expanded our knowledge of the *modus operandi* of NET. It had also confirmed that the various parameters of current which I had discovered by trial and error over the previous several years to be optimum in treating patients, were in most cases the same parameters found to be optimum in detoxifying rats from various drugs, in a series of controlled experiments. Rapid detoxification was a consistent finding in all the rat experiments throughout the four years, *provided the correct parameters were used.*[45, 46, 47]

No work has yet been done, to my knowledge, on the effects of NET in acute drug overdosage in humans, but I hypothesise that it could be as valuable a tool in overdose with, for example, sleeping pills and barbiturates, as a naloxone injection is in patients unconscious from opioid overdosage (they regain consciousness a few minutes after injection). However, our rat work confirmed that each different group of psychoactive drugs requires a different stimulation frequency to achieve maximum rapidity of detoxification (unpublished observations). We also observed widely separated non-linear 'windows' of significant frequencies, as others have discovered, for example, in the frequency-dependent release of substance P from the myenteric plexus in vitro.[112]

As already mentioned the American research physicist Dr Stubbs declared:

> The language of the brain is frequency. Some of the implications of this statement are beginning to be understood. Some observations we do not yet understand. When we learn to speak the frequency language of the brain, we may begin to understand what it is saying.[301]

Scientists in various university laboratories have produced work which substantiates such statements, in particular the frequency-dependent release of transmitter substances.[32, 78, 157] For example, noradrenaline release from individual nerve cells in culture can be potentiated by electromagnetic field (EMF) stimulation at 500 Hz[88] and the effects of dopamine agonists, antagonists and of uptake inhibitors on dopamine and acetylcholine release are highly dependent on the frequency of stimulation used.[77] Reports have also been published in Sweden[287] and Norway[162] describing frequency-dependent effects on pain relief in patients being treated by electrical stimulation for chronic pain.

Again, in measuring the effects of pulsing electromagnetic fields (PEMFs) on peripheral nerve regeneration, 15 Hz gave results only slightly better than controls, whereas 72 Hz 'produced a significant and consistent effect on distal migration of axons'.[175]

Liver function

It is well known that alcohol abuse damages the liver; it is less well known that many drug abusers, even those who have never contracted hepatitis, also have damaged livers. After NET treatment, liver function improved rapidly in patients with hepatic insufficiency. We also demonstrated in rats that hepatic enzyme activity is enhanced by NET,[48] and, in a small sample of healthy, non-smoking humans, hepatic efficiency improved (unpublished observations). And as Dr Robert Moore, Professor of Psychiatry at the University of California, expressed it, 'Detoxification of alcohol is a function of the liver, not doctors or hospitals or detoxification centers'.[215]

Endogenous opioids

The basic relationship between heroin addiction and endogenous opioid systems has been described in Chapter 7. Since the discovery of endorphins in Aberdeen in 1975 by Professor Kosterlitz, many physicians and scientists the world over have shown an association between addictions and altered levels of various neurohormones and neurotransmitters. Conflicting and complex results have emerged, but some reasonably well-established relationships can be briefly described.

The opioid peptides, which consist mainly of the enkephalins, the endorphins and the dynorphins, have the most obvious association with addiction to heroin or other pain-killers. Over 20 different natural substances in this group have now been isolated, as well as three different types of receptor to which they attach,[177] perhaps more. They have different functions in the body but their main function is controlling pain and emotion – as does the exogenous heroin – and *level of motivation for various kinds of purposeful behaviour.*[33]

β-endorphin, self-administered by rats in doses far below that required for an analgesic response, acts as a positive reinforcer of the reward mechanism, similar to heroin injections.[330] An interesting recent discovery is that the enkephalins, as well as their precursors, are localized in the chromaffin granules of the adrenal medulla and may be secreted into the bloodstream (where they have a very short lifetime) during stimulation of the adrenal medulla; the significance of this is still uncertain.[184]

It is hypothesized that in heroin addiction, constant occupation of the opioid receptors by heroin causes the brain's feedback mechanism to reduce the activity of the endorphinergic and enkephalinergic neurons.[144] This feedback effect has been demonstrated in rats made morphine dependent for over one month. Certain parts of their brains showed a 50 per cent decrease in β-endorphin, met-enkephalin and adrenocorticotropic hormone (ACTH), and the plasma β-endorphin levels were also greatly reduced.[117]

Likewise, in one study in humans, the plasma β-endorphin levels in heroin-addicted men were only 345 pg per ml, as against 1,024 pg per ml in non-addicted men under control conditions.[131] The results in methadone addicts are conflicting, but Dr Mark Gold, a New Jersey researcher, reports that more methadone addicts than controls, in his series, had no detectable β-endorphin.[117]

The acute withdrawal symptomatology on abrupt cessation of opioid use could be explained by a rebound hyperactivity of the locus coeruleus, the area which has one of the highest concentrations of endorphins and opioid receptors in the brain. The locus coeruleus hyperactivity evokes increased activity of its norepinephrine cells, producing anxiety and panic, with no endorphin production to balance or brake the norepinephrine overactivity.[117]

ENDORPHINS AND ELECTROSTIMULATION

In pages 127–29 of Chapter 7 the efficacy of electrical stimulation in reducing pain, and its association with the endorphin system, has been briefly described. Its use in drug addiction, as well as its varied biochemical effects, has also been reported in medical literature.

Electro-acupuncture of addicted mice with naloxone-precipitated withdrawal diminished withdrawal symptoms and led to an increase in brain, but not plasma, β-endorphin[340] (the relationship between plasma and CSF levels of the opioid peptides has yet to be established). However, in another series of experiments, drug-termination induced withdrawals, without naloxone, did show increases of both β-endorphin and met-enkephalin in the plasma of addicted rats when treated by electro-acupuncture, which also reduced withdrawal scores to −85 per cent.[349]

Heroin addicts given electro-acupuncture showed amelioration of withdrawal symptoms and a simultaneous increase of met-enkephalin, which had been low before treatment, but not of β-endorphin, in the CSF.[57] If it is true, as Dr Sidney Cohen of UCLA speculates, that 'individuals with low enkephalin levels might be susceptible to depression',[62] this increase in enkephalin could explain the mood elevation that has been consistently noted in our NET patients.

On the other hand, electro-acupuncture given to patients with recurrent pain produced increased levels of β-endorphin but not of met-enkephalin.[58] Swedish workers have likewise found increased CSF levels of endorphins after electro-acupuncture.[288] These findings suggest that the mechanisms involved in the relief of addictions differ from those in pain relief.

Indeed, our own research in rats suggests that stimulation of the endorphins is closely frequency-related, and that the effects of only lower frequencies are endorphin mediated, since prior administration of naloxone at low frequencies negates detoxifying effects.[47]

However, an intriguing finding was that naloxone actually potentiates detoxification from barbiturates at higher frequencies.[47] Also, rat experiments suggest that the site of application of current may be of less importance with high frequency stimulation (500 Hz) than in low frequency (10 Hz) stimulation.[46] However there are risks in using high frequency in humans which must be well understood by the practitioner.

Perhaps the most fascinating experiment is that of Dr Salar of Italy. Measurement of opioid peptides is both easier and more accurate in CSF than in plasma, but few doctors are prepared to subject patients to lumbar puncture for the sake of biochemical measurements alone. However, Dr Salar had thirteen patients with a chronic CSF fistula, and thus frequent CSF measurements could be performed without any traumatic procedure. None of these patients had pain problems. He gave them electrical stimulation through skin electrodes at 40 to 60 Hz and their CSF showed a consistent rise in β-endorphin levels, starting 20 minutes after the beginning of stimulation, peaking after 45 minutes of stimulation and returning to baseline levels, after 90 minutes. Measurements were made by column chromatography and radioimmunoassay (RIA). He theorizes that after one hour the stores of endorphins are depleted, but a suspension of electrotherapy allows recovery to the previous condition, that is, in non-pain, non-addicted subjects.[278] Dr Huda Akil, one of America's foremost researchers in opioid peptides, has reported that localized electrical brain stimulation in patients whose chronic pain was relieved by this technique, likewise had increased enkephalin-like material or immunoreactive β-endorphin in their CSF.[7, 133]

Serotonin

It is possible that NET may also be partly mediated through serotonergic pathways.[17] This could partly explain the strongly positive mood effects that we see in NET patients, often quite early in the 10-day course of treatment, although at the moment there is no conclusive evidence to corroborate this hypothesis.

It has been found that patients with either chronic pain or depression have low central serotonin levels[295] and depressed patients low levels of platelet serotonin.[280] In addition, an association has been demonstrated between suicidal behaviour and low CSF levels of hydroxyindole acetic acid (HIAA – the main metabolite of serotonin).[20, 42] Therefore, the risk of suicide is considered to be greater in those with low serotonin levels.[329] It has also been suggested that serotonin deficiencies may be a factor in obesity, though the possible effect of NET in this area has yet to be investigated.

Electrical stimulation through surgically implanted electrodes has been shown to increase serotonin (5HT) synthesis.[79, 123] In our own research with rats given acute injections of hexobarbital (which in itself decreases the turnover of serotonin in the brain[213]), NET significantly increased the serotonin turnover in the brain compared to the rats in the control group - who also took almost twice as long to recover from the hexobarbital anaesthesia as did NET-treated rats.[45] Electro-acupuncture given to patients with chronic pain has also been shown to raise the platelet serotonin significantly.[199]

In addition, some of my patients have volunteered the information that their chronically cold hands or feet became warm while they were receiving NET for other conditions. A hypothesis was presented in 1983 that transcutaneous electrical treatment giving relief to cases of peripheral ischaemia (poor blood supply to the hands or feet, making them chronically cold) in Raynaud's disease and diabetic polyneuropathy, may act through a central effect on serotonin, since the vasodilation was antagonized by a central serotonin blocker.[165]

In withdrawal from dependency on ethanol (alcohol), morphine, nicotine and phenobarbitone, there is inhibition of serotonin synthesis in the rat brain.[23] Additionally, human chronic alcoholics, during a phase of abstinence, have reduced CSF serotonin.[329] The effects of NET stimulation on serotonergic function may provide a tentative explanation as to why alcohol patients respond so positively to NET.

ACTH

Adrenocorticotropic hormone (ACTH) is another substance which appears to be of clinical importance in drug withdrawal, particularly in the chronic abstinence syndrome. ACTH and β-endorphin have a common precursor, pro-opiocortin (POMC),[273] and they are secreted concomitantly by the pituitary gland.[125] ACTH is released into the circulation in response to stress, and this in turn rapidly stimulates the cortex of the adrenal gland to secrete more cortisol. Both ACTH and cortisol levels have been found to be diminished in the plasma of heroin[131] and methadone[115] addicts. Likewise, there is a low central nervous noradrenaline turnover in high alcohol consumers during long term abstinence.[36]

When Dr Gold and his colleagues tested the cortisol response to an intravenous injection of naloxone, normal subjects showed a consistently brisk rise in plasma ACTH, β-endorphin and cortisol levels, but methadone addicts had a significant suppression of the cortisol response.[117] Other researchers have confirmed these findings, although some consider this lack of response to be due to a primary rather than a secondary hypoadrenalism.[254] This diminished function of the adrenal glands in methadone addicts could explain their 'fatiguability, weakness, anorexia, weight loss, depression and gastrointestinal dysfunction' which 'often persist long after detoxification and are commonly associated with recidivism'.[82]

Stress increases cortisol levels, but rats treated by NET while subjected to restraint stress had less than half the cortisol levels of the control group, suggesting that electro-stimulation significantly ameliorates the effects of stress. (Paradoxically, mixed function oxidase activity, which increases in response to both stress and cortisol, was increased in this experiment, along with the decreased cortisol, instead of being decreased.[48]) Likewise, in both heroin-addicted subjects and normal controls given electro-acupuncture at 125 Hz, the plasma ACTH and cortisol levels were reduced.[341]

Another finding was that while low frequency (10 Hz) and high frequency (500 Hz) both significantly reduced the detoxification time in rats anaesthetized by hexobarbital, the plasma corticosterone levels were markedly decreased by low frequency and increased by high frequency NET.[47] This latter effect could explain the rapid recovery in NET-treated patients of the drug-induced hypoadrenalism, as evidenced by the rapid disappearance of their lethargy - no other type of withdrawal diminishes this persistent lethargy - and the increase in optimism, in contrast to the usual depression.

Alcohol withdrawal

The relationship between the endorphins and alcoholism remains unclear, although some reports have shown that a certain class of opioid receptors is reduced in number by chronic alcohol use in rats.[12, 149] Some researchers have claimed that the body's natural production of endorphins or enkephalins is absent or diminished in alcohol as well as narcotic addiction.[129]

Both in vitro and in vivo studies have shown that ethanol specifically interacts with opioid receptor sites. In rats, only acute ethanol ingestion stimulates striatal met-enkephalin release; after chronic ethanol consumption, diminished enkephalin release can be detected in rat striatum.[196]

The picture in alcohol is certainly more complicated. Researchers in Queen Charlotte's Hospital in London think they may be on the track of the elusive natural ligand for the benzodiazepine receptor (the 'Valium receptor').[59] They have extracted naturally occurring material from human urine which, when given to volunteers, caused uncontrollable panic and required Valium to calm them down. This substance was christened 'tribulin' by Professor Merton Sandler. Further research showed that this material can act directly at the benzodiazepine receptor[113] and Professor Sandler hypothesises that tribulin and the endogenous equivalent of Valium act to form a natural dynamic balance between overstimulation and dopiness. Tribulin appears to be connected with panic, stress and anxiety symptoms, is abnormally high in alcoholic withdrawal (as well as in Valium withdrawal)[247] and does not fall to normal in alcoholics until 6 months after they stop drinking.[318] However, this work has not yet been corroborated by any other group.

GABA

Acute reduction in gamma-aminobutyric acid (GABA) function has also been noted in withdrawal from anxiolytic agents such as ethanol, barbiturates and benzodiazepines.[208]

Impairment of GABA transmission produces a variety of seizure disorders, including grand-mal fits, and modifies the acetylcholine and monoamine systems to promote sleep disorders and delirium - all symptoms seen in withdrawal from these anxiolytic drugs.[74] Again, this is of interest since GABA may be involved in stimulation-produced analgesia (SPA).[195]

Biochemical effects of exercise

Since 1973, we have encouraged our patients to exercise hard (or do outdoor physical work) from the start of their NET treatment; the beneficial effects were evident, despite the effort of will required to do this in the first few days. It has now been discovered that such hard exercise is a natural stimulant of the endorphin system, so we have made this an integral part of both the initial and long-term treatment.

After a long-distance run by trained runners, it was shown that plasma levels of β-endorphin-like immunoreactivity, growth hormone, ACTH and prolactin were all elevated. To further demonstrate that the endorphin system was involved, the runners were given an injection of naloxone after plasma measurements were taken at the end of the run. It was noted, amongst other findings, that 'naloxone attenuated the elevation in joy and euphoria ratings' that were experienced by all runners![155]

This resembles an experiment described by Professor Avram Goldstein of Stanford University in a lecture I attended in California. He gave naloxone to volunteers while they were listening to music which gave *them* particular pleasure, whether it was rock or classical. The naloxone took away the pleasurable experience of the music!

Another series of experiments was carried out with 18 young volunteers who had not previously engaged in regular exercise, and were then given regular training in running. Plasma β-endorphin-like immunoreactivity showed significant increases above basal, reaching peak values at 120 minutes, that is, at the end of the exercise period; the peak concentrations varied from 40 to 1,706 ng per litre (normal values are 10 to 80 ng per litre or less). Likewise, plasma met-enkephalin levels reached a peak of 1,063 ng per litre - over five times the upper limit of normal.[143] Several other similar investigations have been recorded in the literature.

NET, biochemistry and stress

Over 40 neurotransmitters have now been discovered.[153] While altered levels of these substances in any disease are very significant, it is often difficult to know if the change is cause, or effect, or merely part of a chain reaction. The same is true of NET stimulation which alters levels of some neurotransmitters. However, stimulation of hormone and neurotransmitter production appears to be just as dependent on the correct choice of current parameters as it is in detoxification from substance abuse. I am continuing to research these mechanisms.

Meanwhile, the effects of NET on stress were important and

encouraging to me, first, because they confirmed my own clinical findings with NET over the years, and also because of the scale of the stress problem worldwide and the significant part it played in addictions and other diseases. According to Dr Hans Selye, an endocrinologist known for his pioneering studies of the effects of stress on the human body, even such illnesses as arthritis, heart disease, kidney disease and other circulatory disturbances can often be traced to an overproduction of adrenal hormones due to stress. He states that:

> The apparent cause of illness is often an infection, an intoxication, nervous exhaustion, or merely old age, but actually a breakdown of the hormonal mechanism seems to be the most ultimate cause of death in man ... People could live past 100 by understanding and conquering stress, by taking it into our hands and examining its clinical and psychological properties. Stress has got such properties, and they can be measured.[283]

From the preliminary results of our research, therefore, it appeared that with the successful achievement of addiction detoxification we might be opening the door to a revolutionary approach to treatment for other hitherto intractable human diseases.

Statistical survey of NET

My other area of research was a critical analysis of the clinical effects of NET in a variety of conditions. The following is a summary of the basic findings in addiction to all the main groups of psychoactive drugs. More details are available in the *Journal of Bioelectricity*.[242]

In May 1984, a statistical survey of patients treated in England from 1973 to 1980 was published and is briefly described here. It was funded partly by the British Medical Association, and includes a follow-up of 186 addicts up to eight years after their treatment by NET (130 on various drugs, 30 on alcohol, and 26 on cigarettes).

A detailed analysis is given of the effects of NET on addictions (treatment for other conditions is excluded from this survey) in our clinic from January to December 1980 – funded specifically for a larger-scale clinical trial of NET. It was staffed by qualified nurses who had been trained in NET and in the recording of assessment charts. Patients signed an informed consent form after the treatment had been explained in detail by a doctor, in the presence of the next-of-kin/friend. There was no selection of patients except for the exclusion of any suspected of having an underlying psychosis, since there were no facilities for dealing with such conditions.

Detailed data on the immediate effects of NET are presented only for that one year when nursing staff graded and recorded each patient's progress; these findings closely reflect the results of the previous six years, although improvements in techniques and instrumentation were constantly being introduced.[237] There were no control groups, but the majority of patients were their own controls; nearly all had made at least one attempt, and usually many, to stop their addiction with or without assistance.

Patients' self-ratings were recorded with respect to quality of sleep and overall abstinence syndrome (AS). Records were kept of the time taken to fall asleep, the number of hours of sleep and the overall quality of sleep on a four-point scale, as estimated both by night-nurse and patient.

Additional symptoms more specific to alcohol than other drugs - such as tremor and DTs - were recorded but not charted. Weight was taken daily; temperature, pulse, respirations and blood pressure were recorded twice daily, but apart from a brief and mild weight loss, the pattern detailed by Kolb and Himmelsbach in their classic description of the physiological signs in 'abrupt withdrawal' from opiates, did not occur.[174]

A random selection of urines was tested by a government laboratory. However, we observed that even when no other symptom or sign of withdrawal was present, pupil dilatation, to some extent and often to maximum size, was not counteracted by NET; the pupil size was therefore recorded four times daily as a regular check for opioid use after admission.

The following graphs give an outline of the effects of NET on various withdrawal symptoms. Results for individual drugs could not be exactly analysed because so few patients were using only one drug. On average, each patient at time of admission was taking three different drugs every day.

Figure 8.1 shows the amount of withdrawal symptoms experienced by 102 people suffering from addiction to various drugs, alcohol and cigarettes, as recorded by specially trained nurses four times daily. For each symptom which presented, it was graded on a 1-4 scale, 1 indicating the slightest and 4 the greatest severity of

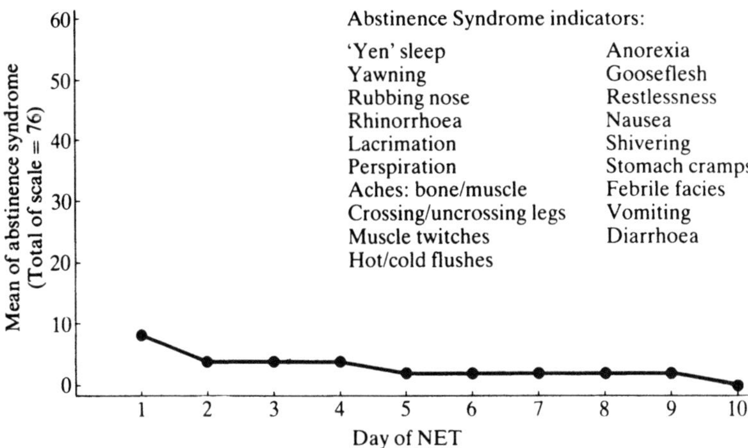

Figure 8.1 Mean of daily means of the abstinence syndrome for all addictions combined ($n = 102$), January–December 1980, based on Himmelsbach's categorization.[174] Each of the 19 signs and symptoms were recorded on a 0–4 point scale, totalling a possible 76, 1 indicating the slightest possible symptom and 4 the greatest severity of the symptom. No patient was graded 4 (the worst) in every indicator simultaneously. The dominant abstinence syndrome indicators varied between patients.

that symptom. If a patient had every possible symptom to the most severe degree, a total of 76 points would have been recorded. This, however, never happened, because all drugs were totally stopped on admission and NET started immediately.

The highest average, in 102 patients, was nine points out of the possible 76, confirming that NET is remarkably successful in reducing withdrawal suffering, without the need for any other drugs.

All patients were initially sceptical of NET's ability to prevent their suffering during the withdrawal period. When recidivist patients undergo a second treatment, this fear of suffering is removed because of their previous experience of NET and the confidence thus gained. Figure 8.2 illustrates how actual symptoms are diminished when the fear of suffering has been removed.

Craving, anxiety and lethargy are three withdrawal symptoms that are not relieved by any form of withdrawal treatment other than NET. Because of their significance, craving and anxiety were recorded separately for 102 consecutive patients. Figure 8.3 shows the rapid decrease in both craving and anxiety experienced by the second day of NET compared to the day of admission. By the

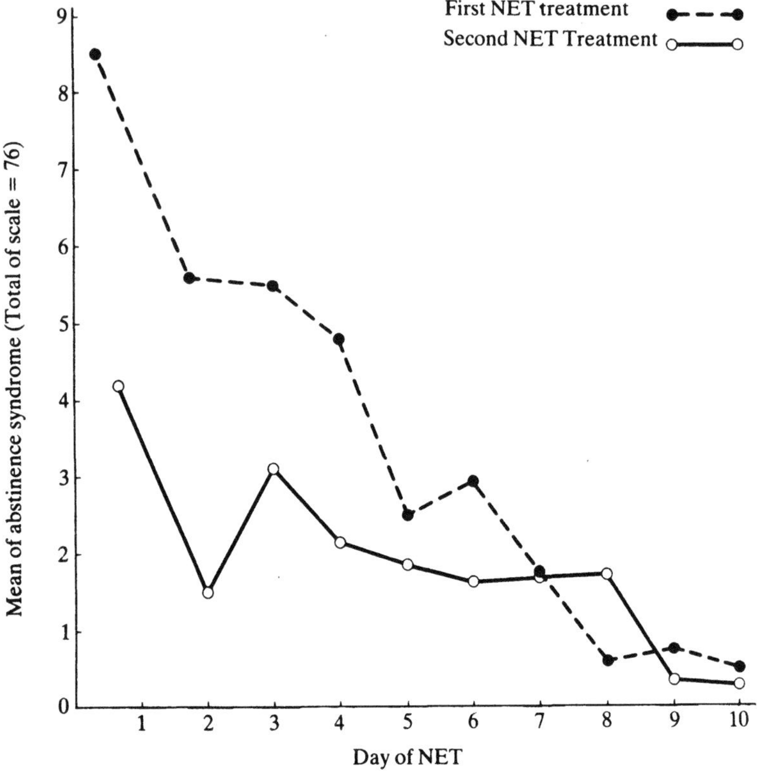

Figure 8.2 Comparison of the abstinence syndrome for 10 subjects on their first treatment by NET, and on re-admission for a second treatment by NET. The vertical axis has been shortened from 76 points to 9 to highlight the differences between reactions to the first and second treatments.

tenth day of NET, 95 per cent of the patients claimed they were free of craving and 75 per cent that they were free of anxiety.

FOLLOW-UP

Before 1980, any patients who were willing to accept rehabilitation after NET had to be transferred to some therapeutic community (TC). Because so few would accept this, from January to December 1980, during the clinic research period, patients were encouraged to remain in the clinic for an additional stay of up to 30 days after NET (this is designated as days of rehabilitation in the results).

Questionnaires were sent by post, but some patients who did not reply were instead interviewed by staff. The questionnaires con-

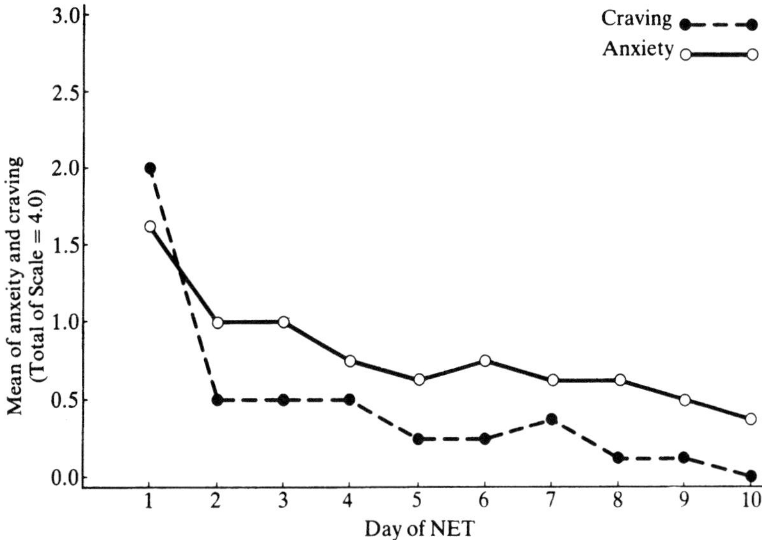

Figure 8.3 Mean of daily means for each subject for craving and anxiety ($n = 102$). Recordings were made four times daily for days 1 to 5 and twice daily for days 6 to 10. In each condition 4 represents the maximum of the symptom and 0 the least.

sisted mainly of multiple outcome variables. Because of inadequate funding, there was no follow-up of the 95 drug addicts, 32 alcoholics and 15 smokers who came for a single preliminary interview but did not return for treatment, for their own financial or other reasons.

The follow-up questionnaires showed that craving tended to recur when patients returned to their former life-situation, but for 80 per cent it had finally disappeared within four months of NET. There are no known studies concerning the time it takes for drug craving to disappear after standard treatments, but methadone addicts in a drug-free TC indicated that it took at least 10 months to diminish and this while still resident in the TC.

INSOMNIA

After withdrawal from heroin and amphetamines, it takes two months for a normal sleep pattern to return,[185, 230] up to four months after barbiturate withdrawal[166] and probably several weeks after stopping alcohol. The effect of NET, without hypnotics, on the sleep pattern is perhaps the most clear and impressive evidence of rapid physiological recovery, the majority regaining a normal, drug-free sleep pattern between the third and ninth nights of NET.[241] A specific frequency of current was found to stop persistent nightmares.

Most patients were willing to accept a drug-free programme. In only a few cases was sedation necessary for the patient's well-being. Only oral paraldehyde was used because it would guarantee a full night's sleep without risk of overdosage; in addition, the foul taste and after-effects ensured no repeat requests.

CONVULSIONS

Convulsions occur in withdrawal from a wide range of psychotropic drugs,[74] e.g. persistent convulsions were reported in two infants born of mothers under treatment with the tricyclic antidepressant clomipramine.[73] Even in gradual withdrawal from diazepam (Valium) at an average daily dose of only 10 mg or lorazepam (Ativan) at 4 mg, 2.5 per cent of the patients in Tyrer's series of 40 suffered epileptic seizures.[324] Few in the NET series used such small dosages.

Out of 126 patients who admitted to using drugs with the potential for causing withdrawal convulsions, 60 (47.6 per cent) took above-maximum therapeutic doses. Seven (5.5 per cent) had seizures. No patient had more than one brief seizure except for one, treated in 1977, who had previously suffered multiple convulsions. He had been taking 1,000 mg pentobarbital (Nembutal, 10 capsules), 1,000 mg chlormethiazole (Heminevrin, 10 capsules) and 60 mg flurazepam (Dalmane, four capsules) daily for three years, and was on phenytoin (Epanutin, an anti-convulsant) on admission. His phenytoin was continued, the pentobarbital was slowly withdrawn, yet he had multiple seizures, hallucinations and delusions. In contrast, among the patients treated in 1980 who had only one brief convulsion and whose drugs had been totally stopped on admission, was one who had been taking 5,000 mg Tuinal (50 capsules) daily for 6 months, in addition to 26 tablets of paracetamol (Panadol - for excruciating headaches), 2 g heroin and 3 g cocaine; his headaches also disappeared completely with NET.

Only two patients had alcohol withdrawal convulsions, although 69 per cent of alcoholics treated were taking a hypnosedative or tranquillizer regularly; in both cases, the convulsions were hypoglycaemic.

DELIRIUM TREMENS

No patient experienced DTs and none had hallucinations or delusions except for the one case described above, who was given a gradual withdrawal from barbiturates.

LONG-TERM PHYSICAL EFFECTS

The replies regarding post-NET health, including those referring to non-drug conditions (this review deals only with addictions), reveal no illness which could have resulted from NET, including those receiving long-term treatment for chronic pain. Seventy-five per cent reported overall improvement in health, whether or not there was a relapse in the addiction.

DEATHS

There were eight reported deaths (4.3 per cent) over an eight-year period, all drug addicts. The average time between NET and death was 22 months, only one being less than one year. None were associated with NET and two were apparently unrelated to drugs. One was a suicide and three were not re-addicted but died in their sleep or drowned in their bath after a single episode of heroin combined with alcohol.

This 6.1 per cent death rate (out of 130 drug addicts treated) is disappointingly high, even though it compares favourably with the 15 per cent recorded in a representative sample of 128 patients of London drug dependence clinics over 10 years;[297, 344] or 20.5 per cent in an eleven-year follow-up of all 83 addicts attending another clinic in 1971[71] (in both cases, all were using drugs at the time of death); or 23 per cent in New York over 20 years.[327] In 1981, it was estimated that the known addict mortality rate in England was 27 per thousand addicts *per year*.[62]

DROP-OUT RATE (DOR)

This is probably the most significant indicator both of patient acceptability of any treatment and of clinical effectiveness. In this series, the DOR over seven years was 1.6 per cent. The 10 per cent who said they would not wish to have NET again did not object to the NET per se but indicated that the treatment they needed was psycho-therapeutic.

Other programmes report higher rates of DOR; for example, the USA Drug Abuse Reporting Program (DARP), mostly opioid users, records 71 per cent over three years (i.e. excluding their control group, although their criteria of 'drop-out' is not clear; our criterion was failure to complete detoxification)[286] and the drop-out rate in Tyrer's series (low dosage diazepam or lorazepam) 45 per cent.[324] The well-known Haight-Ashbury Drug Clinic in San Francisco use electro-acupuncture effectively, yet there is a 90 per cent DOR from the 21-day treatment; but of those who completed the course, 30 per cent were drug-free at the end of one year.[152]

RECIDIVISM

A low recidivist rate and improved quality of life are the best indicators of diminution of the chronic withdrawal syndrome. Because of insufficient staff and funding, only 50 per cent of patients treated over seven years could be traced. Despite this low response rate, the NET drug-free rate of 80.3 per cent (for drug addicts only) is encouraging. De Leon reports of Phoenix House in New York that 'over 50 per cent of those who had remained a year or longer in residence were successful across 5 years of follow-up' but his criteria of success included methadone maintenance. He goes on to say that 'when effectiveness is defined in terms of heroin or methadone abstinence, less than 10 per cent are judged successful, 10 years after treatment'.[86]

Another large-scale measurement of drug treatment results in USA concerns a residential treatment programme, managed largely by medical specialists, under the auspices of New York State's Narcotic Addiction Control Commission. They reported in 1979 that 'of the 5172 people who entered the program, 141 were drug-free at the end of eighteen months. Thus the program had a cure rate of 3 percent.'[223]

Surveys worldwide have shown that 'success' is directly related to 'time spent in treatment', usually in some form of therapeutic community (TC)[285]; the majority insist on a 'minimum residency of 18-24 months'[86]. In contrast, only 42 per cent of NET patients had any such residency and these for an average stay of only 16 days. Analysis of our figures showed that the eventual outcome was unrelated to the time spent in 'rehabilitation'.[242]

It is realized that many who are treated by NET still need the help of a TC or other support system, but the time required is considerably less if preceded by NET, perhaps partly because of their sense of physical well-being. In addition, there are many drug addicts and alcoholics who refuse hospitalization, let alone long-term residency. Thus the short duration of NET may encourage many who otherwise would make no attempt to discontinue drugs or alcohol.

Of respondents to follow-up, 17 per cent had one treatment after NET (a second NET or other hospital treatment) and 1 per cent had two treatments. In contrast, in a 1982 US Government survey, from 26 per cent to 43 per cent had repeat treatments *every year* (the number of treatments per year is not stated) after the initial treatment, for up to six years.[316]

Of NET drug-free, 23.5 per cent admit to having used alcohol as a substitute for their drug/s, but only temporarily in every case, an unusually low incidence of alcohol substitution. The same USA survey reported 60 per cent as drinking moderately or heavily three to six years after treatment.[316]

Other data from the NET questionnaires indicate a consistent improvement in quality of life and relationships, and some reductions in alcohol, marijuana and cigarette use. The re-addicted also showed some improvement in these areas; in addition, 35 per cent remained addiction-free for more than six months after NET and 76 per cent were using less of their substance of abuse than before NET.

Twenty-eight (21.5 per cent) of the drug addicts treated by NET were registered with drug dependency units and 10 of these responded to follow-up. Only 6 per cent of drug-free were registered, against 54 per cent of the re-addicted. Although not statistically significant, this would tend to confirm the belief of many drug addicts that if they register, they 'will never stop drug abuse because it is so easy to get the drugs'.

Of the drug-free respondents, 62 per cent have occasionally experimented with heroin after NET but discontinued it spontaneously because they found it 'unsatisfactory'. In contrast, when they had stopped heroin previously by any other method, a single episode was sufficient to re-addict them.

This unexpected reaction could be due to long-term beneficial effects of NET. Some addicts with the ability to analyse their responses to drugs said that they wanted to experience heroin again in order to prove to themselves that the cycle of indulgence and addiction, in the sense of bondage, was really broken.

A 20-year-old girl wrote describing her relapse, which happened five weeks after completing NET:

I believe that without NET there would be no way that I would have stopped using heroin. The difference I feel between NET and being given methadone or any heroin substitute is that with NET it is an almost immediate detoxification - there is no long battle lasting for months on end.

I think at this moment the reason why I took it again was that I had totally given up on myself. Unlike before, I felt 'uncomfortable' all the time I was under the influence and I was also sick, something that rarely happened before NET. It lasted about a week - then I told my employer. I haven't done any more heroin or any other drug since that day and I felt no after effects.

I now have no craving whatsoever - in fact I am frightened of the control I can now see that heroin had over me ... It was a great help to me going back to my parents and telling them the truth because in doing this I felt I had nothing to hide anymore from anyone.

And a cogent description from a 34-year-old married man with children:

You correctly predicted a relapse and though it was physically soothing it was also acrid and hollow, sheltering from a cold rain in a cave full of bat dung. The reunion was brief and any pleasure defeated by the pain and confusion it caused my patient loved ones. It was like looking for a tarnished penny in a gold mine, more wasted time and strength.

My greatest problem has been in giving myself to the ones who need me. Every touch is like a visit to the dentist, unpleasant enough to provoke gnawing impotent guilt and yet simultaneously rewarding and healing. Bursting with metaphors I want to believe that the destination is worth the voyage.

III PSYCHO-THERAPEUTIC PROBLEMS AND PSYCHO-SPIRITUAL SOLUTIONS

Chapter 9
Addicts' need for psychotherapy

> Heroin, I love you. You are God. Heroin, without you, I am nothing. Heroin, my one, true, only *real* LOVE! I love you with every cell of my being. You take me to hell and I love you for it. You present a phony heaven and I adore you the more. You fill my mind. Yes, I love you, and I hate you with a hatred so deep, so deep a thousand worlds could burn in the strength of my hate.

These are the words of an addict who wrote to me recently, describing what heroin addiction means to him.

> I had become addicted to those five or ten minutes of 'kingliness' that came with the first sniff and which I would madly attempt to repossess for however many frantic hours my supply of coke would last me. I spent seven days and seven nights without sleep, chasing that elusive euphoria. It was this mad decline of my rush into cocaine that quite surely led me to heroin itself.
>
> Here perhaps lies one of the deepest keys to why I became an addict. I was always an inward-turning, self-absorbed, self-centred person, and one of the great dangers for the spiritual seeker is the possibility that intense self-study, necessary enough for the attainment of true self-awareness, not become instead a deep narcism (sic). In my case, narcism won over in the subtle struggle. Instead of a dissolution of the ego there came a dissolution of the will and a fortifying of the ego.
>
> However, for all addicts, there comes the Rude Awakening. Then the full horror of addiction to heroin becomes only too evident. The deeper the psychic, spiritual deprivation experienced, the more powerful becomes the terrific struggle, the tug-of-war to, on the one hand, break loose for ever from the vicious cycle, or to continue to sink deeper and deeper into the mire that the drug has dumped you in. The habit of living a painless, careless, somnolent life is harder to break than the mere physical suffering . . .

Dealing with underlying problems

One of the problems with the rapid detoxification produced by NET is that patients are suddenly faced again with all the problems that led to addiction. On the fourth day, experienced addicts know that if they haven't had any withdrawal symptoms, they aren't going to have any. With their own endorphins flooding their systems once again, they generally experience an immense euphoria, thinking 'At last I've got this thing licked.'

This rapid return to alertness and responsiveness is one of the most impressive features of NET, contrasting strongly with the lethargy and depression which accompany all other forms of treatment.[15, 53, 115, 116, 337] Friends and relatives often comment on how rapidly a patient returns to the kind of person he or she was before going on drugs.

And the rehabilitative process has to begin on the second or third day because the addicts become responsive to counselling with unusual rapidity. This is when the really hard work begins - and it *is* very hard work. Coming off drugs by NET, the mind becomes clear, with no physiological distraction, for the first time since starting drug use. This makes not only the pleasure more intense - but also pain.

The most important element in NET is that it appears to remove completely the chronic withdrawal syndrome which with other ways of stopping drugs can go on for many months, up to a year and a half, making them feel not necessarily ill but just not well. Because NET makes them feel so much better, both physically and emotionally, they should be more able to cope with the problems that lie ahead.

Rehabilitation or revitalization

The second phase of NET treatment is designed to help individuals who are, on the one hand, hoping that they can overcome addiction, but who are at the same time aware of their own total inadequacy in dealing with personal, psychological, social, domestic or spiritual problems.

In my seven-year follow-up, the questionnaires sent to patients contained the following questions - the answers are given here in percentages.[242]

	DRUG OR ALCOHOL FREE (80, 78)	RECIDIVISTS (20, 22)
Relationships with family/spouse:		
Outstanding improvement	67	37
Slight improvement	15	27
The same	18	27
Worse	0	9
Are you more able to cope with the problems of living than previously?		
Much better	68	30
Slightly better	26	20
The same	4	40
Worse	2	10
If you were readdicted and wished to come off, would you do so by NET?		
Yes	89	94
No	11	6

All who said they would not want to use NET again commented that it was not because of NET itself, but because they felt that the treatment they needed was psychological, not physical. But as my husband described in an interview:

> The fourth day is a sixteen-hour one, starting at 8 o'clock in the morning and going right through to 10 or 12 o'clock at night. The addicts have to look at themselves as they have not looked at themselves in years. They are facing a day in which they don't have to try to con husband, wife or friend. They don't have to rip off the police or a garage or pharmacy. They are just sitting, and that hurts.
>
> They've got out of the habit of filling their days with anything constructive, whether it's working, reading, listening to music or whatever. They have sixteen hours of total boredom, in which they are left looking at the problem that they looked at the day they started on drugs. They didn't like themselves back then, they didn't like their lives, parents, home, society, church or God. But they managed to live with all those things as long as they had the chemical. Now that their chemical has been taken away they are brought back to the day in which they first decided to run from their problems.[110]

The anatomy of addiction

To understand why rehabilitation is equally as important as detoxification, addicts, their friends and families must appreciate why the habit developed in the first place, however painful the reading is.

As William Burroughs, the American writer-addict, said, 'The question, of course, could be asked: Why did you ever try narcotics? Why did you continue using it long enough to become an addict? You become a narcotics addict because you do not have strong enough motivations in any other direction. Junk wins by default.'[44]

The problem 'is a problem neither of youth nor one of drugs, but a problem of a whole society and an entire life-style shared by young and old alike' (quoting the evidence of a doctor before a US Senate Committee on the Judiciary, 17 September 1969).

Addiction is a complex problem with roots in the individual, family and society, sometimes coming to the surface early in life and sometimes much later. There is not sufficient evidence to indicate anything so strong as the 'addictive personality' postulated by some psychiatrists. However, one common feature has been found among drug addicts observed in the addiction epidemics in Japan as well as in North America and Britain – an absent, weak, or inadequate father. As one American researcher recently expressed it, a 'weak, ineffectual, non-disciplining or absent father figure (is) found to be the most commonly significant contributing factor in the culture'.[128]

An addict is someone who cannot deal with people or circumstances in his or her immediate environment, because of personal inadequacy. Philosophically, it has been suggested that *adaequatio rei est intellectus* – the understanding of the knower must be adequate to the thing to be known. In everyday terms we are talking about the inability of the individual to cope with family, school, office, workshop, boardroom, household or social occasion without the 'support' of some chemical substance.

Without the cigarette, drink or drug such an individual soon becomes a very anti-social creature, cogently described by one noted authority:

> Addicted patients are asocial, inadequate, immature and unstable. They are selfish and self-centered without interest in the welfare of others and are only concerned with their own problems. Their major

> problem is in their maintenance of the supply of drugs or the immediate gratification of their desire for drugs. They will resort to any means - however unreasonable or dangerous - to satisfy this insistent craving. They have failed to develop normal human relationships and are almost totally without concern for the distress they inflict on their relatives. They lack self-discipline, will-power or ambition and avoid responsibility. They have a low threshold for pain or any form of discomfort, and are unable to tolerate criticism or to bear frustration. Their personal relationships tend to become confined to other members of the drug addicts' world, and thus they become social outcasts and very lonely people.[181]

Incisive as this analysis is, it is still only a superficial description of an addict; it does not penetrate deep enough to provide a true explanation of the problem from which to move towards a possible solution. It is necessary to explore the intricacies of social structures, family relationships and, ultimately, the mind of individual addicts. The whole person must be understood - body, mind, and *spirit* (a dimension rarely acknowledged by psychiatrists, although, significantly, emphasized with a greater measure of success by the more spiritually-oriented Alcoholics Anonymous) in order to reach some understanding of the cause and so begin to develop a cure.

Dr Stanton Peele, in his book *Love and Addiction*, has described it this way:

> An addict is a person who never learns to come to grips with his world, and who therefore seeks stability and reassurance through some repeated, ritualized activity. This activity is reinforced in two ways; first, by a comforting sensation of well-being induced by the drug or other addictive object; second, by the atrophy of the addict's other interests and abilities and the general deterioration of his life situation while he is preoccupied with his addiction. As alternatives grow smaller the addiction grows larger, until it is all there is. A true addict progresses into a monomania, whether the object of addiction is a drug or a lover.[244]

Addiction, therefore, is *alienation* - from parents, or children, or friends, or churches, or God. Addiction is *emptiness* - a vast and tedious apathy, a meaningless continuum, a sense of insignificance, or anonymity, or purposelessness. Addiction is *inadequacy* - in personal relationships, or studies, or employment, or housework; it is inability to perform the smallest responsible task. Addiction is *guilt* - about failure as parent, or child, or husband, or wife, or manager, or employee; as cynic or sycophant, as leader or led, as teacher or student, as artist or artisan, as neighbour or colleague.

Dr Peele expands his definition of an addict:

> In these terms, then, an addiction exists when a person's attachment to a sensation, an object, or another person is such as to lessen his appreciation of and ability to deal with other things in his environment, or in himself, so that he has become increasingly dependent on that experience as his only source of gratification. A person will be predisposed to addiction to the extent that he cannot establish a meaningful relationship to his environment as a whole, and thus cannot develop a fully elaborated life.[244]

In laboratory experiments with rats, some of the complexities of addictions have been observed. Laboratory animals would starve themselves of food rather than cross an electrified grid to reach it; but they would cross that same electrified grid in order to reach a pleasure-stimulus. Other rats were tested with pans of plain water or of heroin solution; the 'leader' rat, and 'lower-rank' rats, after tasting both, kept to the pans of plain water, but the 'middle-rank' rats chose the heroin solution. In yet another experiment, rats which were deprived of all forms of stress gradually lost interest in food, then in sex, and eventually became impotent and died.

Of course, it does not follow *ipso facto* that what is true of rats is also true of humans, but the experimental evidence is at least suggestive: that stress and challenge are necessary elements in life, but to some more than others. Intense stresses cause them to choose the relief of a narcotic, and that, given a choice between food or pleasure, some will opt for pleasure at the risk of possible death. These circumstances were imposed on the rats for the purposes of experiments; humans choose of their own accord to follow similar patterns.

Still other generalizations can be made from observations recorded by those who work with addicts. Seventy per cent of addicts do not have a strong and caring father. Either or both parents of an addict are two to seven times more likely to have been on some kind of mood-altering drugs, such as tranquillizers, than the parents of a non-addict. Most addicts have parents who were either above-average alcohol drinkers, or heavy smokers, or both; most addicts have had anxiety-provoking home circumstances or a history of resorting to legal medications in the past.

Dr David Smith, who founded the Haight-Ashbury Free Medical Clinic in San Francisco in 1967, has stated that the child of an alcoholic parent is 35 times more likely to become addicted himself than the child of a non-alcoholic; this ratio soars to 400 if both parents were alcoholics.[169]

DEPENDENCE NEED NOT BE ADDICTION

A common mistake among those involved with addicts is to confuse 'dependence' with 'addiction'. It is possible to be dependent on a drug and not to be addicted. For example, the diabetic who is dependent on insulin injections and uses a syringe regularly does not become 'addicted' to the drug, with its classic symptoms; nor does the regularity of his insulin injections become the ritualized obsession of the heroin addict.

The distinction is important and involves the dimension of bondage or freedom. Dependence is the relationship between an individual and a drug that is ultimately beneficial (many diabetics on insulin become international athletes); while addiction is the relationship between an individual, a drug and society, that is ultimately destructive (that is, it involves a violation of social norms in patterns of lying, deceit and often stealing). Dependence can be and usually is a healthy experience, as is, for example, the loving inter-dependence between husband and wife, or between children and parents, or between members of a community or church; but when any of these relationships become self-centred and exploitative a new element is introduced, and the relationship becomes one of destructive bondage instead of productive freedom.

ADDICTION IS BONDAGE

Whatever else it is, therefore, addiction is *bondage*. (Actually, that is what the word meant before psychiatrists confused the condition with pseudo-scientific jargon.) The word 'addiction' in English language and literature means 'bondage'. In his book, *Licit and Illicit Drugs*, Edward M. Brecher states this very clearly:

> In Roman law to be addicted meant to be bound over to someone by a judicial sentence; thus the prisoner of war might be addicted to some nobleman or large landowner. In sixteenth century England, the word had the same meaning; thus a serf might be addicted to a master. But Shakespeare and others of his era perceived the marked similarity between this legal form of addiction and a man's bondage

> to alcoholic beverages; they therefore spoke of being 'addicted to alcohol'. Poets also spoke of men 'addicted to vice,' and of women 'addicted to virginity'. Dr Johnson spoke of 'addiction to tobacco,' and John Stuart Mill of 'addiction to bad habits'. The conception of addiction to opium, morphine, and heroin followed quite naturally.[39]

It was mainly because of their inability to understand this important dimension, or unwillingness to address the problem from this standpoint, that many doctors and psychiatrists involved with the treatment of addictions fell into the trap of mechanical mind-tinkering and pill-pushing, with its present disastrous consequences.

One of the world's most famous addicts is the well-known playwright, Jean Cocteau, who wrote a revealing book out of his own experiences. *Opium: The Diary of an Addict* describes his harrowing attempts to come off the drug, and the doctors' attempts to cure him:

> Incredible phenomena are attached to the cure. Medicine is powerless against them, beyond making the padded cell look like a hotel-room and demanding of the doctor or nurse patience, attendance and sensitivity ...
>
> I therefore became an opium addict again because the doctors who cure – one should really say, quite simply, who purge – do not seek to cure the troubles which first cause the addiction ...
>
> After the cure. The worst moment, the worst danger. Health with this void and an immense sadness. The doctors honestly hand you over to suicide.
>
> Now that I am cured, I feel empty, poor, heart-broken and ill.[60]

What a literate, devastating indictment! Other addicts less articulate than Jean Cocteau, but just as aware of the many forms of treatment practised on them, and the varied medications prescribed by doctors, could echo his words: 'Now that I am "cured", I feel empty, poor, heart-broken and ill.' From laudanum to Librium, from morphine to methadone, from alcohol to Ativan, the 'cures' for addiction simply evade the two main questions implicit in the problem of addiction: How may an addict be detoxified from bondage to chemicals? and, How may the underlying emptiness of life be filled?

THE EMPTINESS OF THE ADDICT

In the 1930s Dr Carl Jung, the psychoanalyst, commented: 'About a third of my cases are suffering from no clinically definable neurosis, but from the senselessness and emptiness of their lives. It seems that this can be described as the greatest neurosis of our time.'[160]

This emptiness has not diminished. If anything it has increased, so that Dr Rollo May, a New York psychiatrist, could write in 1969:

> It may seem surprising when I say, on the basis of my own clinical practice, as well as that of my psychological and psychiatric colleagues, that the chief problem of the middle decade of the twentieth century is emptiness ... While one might laugh at the meaningless boredom of people a decade or so ago, the emptiness for many has now moved from the state of boredom to a state of futility and despair which holds promise of dangers.[204]

And the sickness of Western society is described by Paul Tillich in this way:

> A belief breaks down through external events or inner processes: one is cut off from creative participation in a sphere of culture, one feels frustrated about something which one has passionately affirmed, one is driven from devotion to one object to devotion to another and again on to another, because the meaning of each of them vanishes and the creative eros [sic] is transformed into indifference or aversion. Everything is tried and nothing satisfies ... Anxiously one turns away from all concrete contents and looks for an ultimate meaning, only to discover that it was the loss of a spiritual center which took away the meaning from the special contents of the spiritual life ... The anxiety of emptiness drives us to the abyss of meaninglessness.[312]

Thus, when addicts have been detoxified - or, rather, 'dried out', or 'cold-turkeyed', but not really detoxified in the true sense of the term - from their particular chemical of addiction, or de-programmed from their particular ritualized addictive activity, it is glaringly apparent that they are not cured, as Jean Cocteau so graphically stated. They are only removed temporarily from the *consequences* of a particular form of addictive indulgence or behaviour. Unfortunately, it is just at this point of being relieved of a particular consequence that the addict is usually discharged by the doctor or therapist as 'cured' – when both know that the actual cause of addiction has not even been touched.

Needed – a new framework

The real cure of such an individual requires a restructured life, a therapeutic rehabilitation which will provide an adequate framework of values to give meaning to the individual and help towards an understanding of his or her place in society. This framework includes a freedom to choose, a confidence to make the choice, and a responsibility to pay the price of that choice. To do this successfully requires a form of psychotherapy hitherto not known; or, if known, certainly not widely practised. This is elaborated on in Chapter 10.

As has already been noted, emptiness and meaninglessness are spiritual problems, and psychiatry – certainly Freudian psychoanalysis and behaviourism – considers any concern with the spiritual a form of neurosis in itself.

Time magazine, in its 25 April 1983 issue, describes how Dr George Vaillant, a Harvard psychiatrist, evaluates traditional psychiatric approaches to the problem of alcoholism:

> They are nearly useless in dealing with the underlying nature of alcoholism itself. In his book [*The Natural History of Alcoholism: Causes, Patterns, and Paths to Recovery*], Vaillant ruefully describes his own disillusionment with his profession's ability to cope with the disease. 'I was working for the most exciting alcohol program in the world,' he says, 'but the results at the clinic were no better than if the doctors had left the alcoholics alone.'
>
> Other professionals agree with Vaillant's glum assessment. 'We don't do anything adequately,' admits Dr Robert Millman, director of the Alcohol and Drug Abuse Service at Payne Whitney Psychiatric Clinic in New York City.
>
> What about expensive hospital treatment centers, now so fashionable that they have become a growth industry with companies listed on the New York Stock Exchange? Vaillant concludes flatly that they do not work in the long run.

The *Time* article concludes: '... even though it's terribly unscientific, alcoholics usually do seem to need some kind of source of hope and self-esteem, or religious inspiration – whatever you want to call it - and that seems more important than hospital or psychiatric care.'[228]

Dr Vaillant goes on to say:

> Hospitalized patienthood destroys self-esteem, and when hospitalization ceases the patient loses his substitute dependency.
>
> Alcoholics feel defeated, helpless and without ability to change. If their lives are to change, they need hope as much as relief of symptoms ... To change a maladaptive habit ... we cannot 'treat' or compel or reason with the person. Rather, we must change the person's belief systems and then maintain that change ... their habits will follow. In other words, if we can but combine the best placebo effects ... with the best attitude change inherent in the evangelical conversion experience, we may be on our way to an effective alcoholism program ... [All these statistics] bear powerful witness that alcoholics recover not because we treat them but because they heal themselves.[328]

RENEWAL OF VALUES

In an article entitled 'Relief of psychiatric symptoms in evangelical religious sects', which dealt with the emergence of numerous religious sects in the United States and Western Europe in the past decade, the authors concluded:

> Analysis of questionnaires revealed that members of the sects had experienced psychological difficulties prior to conversion. Many had sought professional help for these ... and some even hospitalization ... Members also reported a high incidence of drug use before joining. Approximately one quarter of the respondents in the groups answered in the affirmative to having had serious drug problems in the past ... The proportion who had used drugs of abuse to any extent was much higher than that for a comparable national sample. For example, when compared with a matched group in a national survey about twice as many Divine Light Mission members had ever taken each of the groups of drugs, for example 92 versus 52 per cent for marijuana and 14 versus 6 per cent for heroin ...
>
> However, with conversion a marked change in these parameters was reported. Such change was reflected in neurotic symptom scores noted for the period before joining as compared with those after joining ... *It does indeed appear that the conversion of one's system of beliefs leads to a certain relief of psychological distress* ... The study of charismatic sects teaches us the importance of maintaining a mutually accepted system of norms and beliefs for treatment per-

> sonnel as well as for patients. *If we attempt to effect change without addressing a patient's value systems we risk coming up against impenetrable difficulties.*[109] (my italics)

But it is important to note that, whatever spiritual belief system an individual chooses, it must be adequate to meet, and overcome if necessary, the challenges of the environment in which the individual lives and functions. Otherwise it serves only as a talismanic superstition, and not as an effective value system for change.

In his book, *Drugs: Medical, Psychological and Social Facts*, Peter Lawrie declares:

> Addicts are notoriously resistant to ordinary psychotherapy. One way of looking at this is to observe that analysis depends on communication, on the patient's acceptance of the therapist as a real human being who can have a real effect on him. But the addict's whole life is organised to remove any dependence on humanity: given his drugs, he is self-sufficient, able to generate his own satisfactions and guilts and to live a rich emotional life independent of the outside world. He therefore has no motives for communication when things are going well; when he does present himself for treatment it is often not because he wants to be cured of addiction, but because his addiction is not working as it should. He is a two-time loser who wants to get back to being a one-time loser, not to take the much more perilous step to being an unloser.
>
> The ordinary psychiatric patient is like a burr, offering many hooks to the world and the therapist – often too many; the therapist's best strategy is to stand still and let his patient attach himself as he will. But the addict is like a nut: smooth, with a thick armor. The only hook he offers is his need for drugs, and that can be satisfied in a number of ways. To reach the addict, his shell must be cracked. We might guess that it would be necessary to counter the coercion of opiates with the coercion of therapy.[181]

It is absolutely necessary, therefore, that a satisfactory form of chemical detoxification takes place before any serious attempt at psychotherapy is attempted. What passed for 'detoxification' of addictions was a debasement of the term; addicts might be 'dried out', or 'cold-turkeyed', in a variety of institutions devoted to what was publicized as detoxification, but they were certainly not detoxified in the true sense of the term (which, etymologically speaking, means removing a poisoned arrow).

Dr Avram Goldstein, an international authority on addictions, had made this clear in the quotation mentioned earlier:

> It is still not understood why simple detoxification is so ineffective, but the facts are clear and inescapable ... As I see it, the reason for the dismal failure of detoxification (the majority of subjects relapse before completing the customary 21-to-30-day process) is that the newly detoxified addict, still driven by discomfort, physiologic imbalances, and intense craving, cannot focus attention on the necessary first steps towards rehabilitation, but soon succumbs and starts using heroin again.[119]

If addiction is to be truly cured the emptiness must be filled, meaning must be provided, capacity to love and forgive must be developed, repentance must be encouraged, ability to think must be taught, willingness to take responsibility must be cultivated, hope must be implanted, the seeds of faith and vision must be sown. The individual cannot be left at the mercy of an amorphous, uncaring 'force'. Beyond a bottle, a pill, a powder, an injection, an object, a cause, a ritual, a sensation, all addicts have a spiritual hunger. What they really want is love, or truth, or beauty, or joy, or life, or transcendence, or power – or God. Ultimately God must be recognized as real.

Philosophy of our clinic

To deal only with the detoxification of the addict is irresponsible; and to deal only with the psycho-spiritual problem of the addict is naive. Both aspects of the problem have to be addressed and a system including both detoxification and rehabilitation devised.

As we formulated this in our clinic, we began every morning with our patients spending an hour looking at a newspaper, or reading and thinking about some other material such as the Bible, Gibran's *The Prophet*, or even Karl Marx, if they chose that. The idea was to begin feeding and exercising their minds with tasks of gradually increasing challenge, especially where their mental faculties had been badly eroded by long-term use of drugs.

This was followed by therapy in the form of non-recreational work activities and talks with doctor and counsellor. The afternoons were for tennis, swimming or games, plus individual and group therapy sessions.

No arrangements were made for the employment of patients during a short-term stay, but a list of possible employers and training programs was prepared for later use.

Residents were encouraged to maintain regular contact with the clinic staff following the completion of their inpatient rehabilitation, and a list of families, support groups, churches, and other interested agencies nationwide provided continuing support for former patients. A counselling information package was available to send to all interested employers with their own medical welfare plans.

Believing that addiction has a physiological as well as a psychological derivation, and that the latter, to a great extent, is caused by lack of meaningful relationship with family, relatives, community, or God, and of an inadequate experiential framework to cope with the chosen environment, our philosophy was to treat the whole person, body, mind and spirit, so that not only the chemical or behavioural addiction was cured, but also the underlying cause which produced the addiction in the first place.

Our clinic was not a religious organization. We have treated Muslims, Buddhists, Marxists and Hindus as well as Christians, agnostics and atheists who seek freedom from chemical and behavioural addictions. But it was staffed by personnel who had a wholesome commitment to spiritual ideas and who were professionals, with acknowledged expertise in their fields. There were no psychiatrists on the resident or consultant staff, since addiction is believed to be fundamentally a spiritual problem requiring spiritual solutions which can be more than adequately provided by trained para-professionals with a knowledge and experience of addictions and spiritual values.

My husband and I and our three children lived in the manor house and ate our meals with the patients and staff every day. We considered our observable interaction with each other as a family, and the patients' interaction with a normal family and caring counsellors, to be an important part of the therapeutic process.

SUPERFICIAL RELIGIOUS FORMULAE

Professional religionists with easy formulae have seriously damaged their cause as well as their own reputations with their talismanic versions of Christianity. The difficult process of acquiring spiritual enlightenment has been movingly described by the Russian Marxist-turned-Christian philosopher, Nikolai Berdyaev:

> The suffering that has once been lived through cannot possibly be effaced ... The man who has travelled far in the realms of the spirit, and who has passed through great trials in the cause of his search for truth, will be formed spiritually along lines which must differ altogether from those pertaining to the man who has never shifted his position and to whom new spiritual territories are unknown ... I am enriched by my experience, even if it has been fearful and tormenting, even if to cross the abyss I have been forced to address myself to powers other than human.[31]

MEANINGFUL RELATIONSHIPS

Our own family experience of this in various countries, as we sought to understand and obey the will of God, had given us a unique experience of how to deal with people afflicted with 'emptiness and meaninglessness' in their lives, whether they were drug addicts or not. But with each addicted patient I treated there was no doubt that the root problem was psycho-spiritual and that they despaired of finding ultimate answers. What was there to live for? Why should they come off drugs? How would they cope at home, at work, at play, without them? Who would want to live in such a lousy world without drugs? What was the point of talking about a relationship with a father, a mother, a wife, a husband, a lover, children, friends or God? Who cared whether you lived or died anyway? In their minds the emptiness stretched and deepened into an unbridgeable gulf.

But as we spoke of the spiritual values of love, forgiveness, repentance, mercy, joy, peace, and salvation for all, what began as cynicism from even the most hardened individual moved slowly to wary consideration, and often advanced to tentative or glad acceptance. Living in close contact with others in our clinic, they could see people whose lives did have meaning, who did care. It was not just empty moralizing.

Whenever a patient would come right up front and say, for example, 'The thing is, I just hate my father and can't come to terms with him,' we would try to deal with that individual's problem. We would contact the father, bring parent and child together, and try to point out that forgiveness is an essential part of the healing mechanism. It wasn't enough for parents to want a son or daughter to come off a drug. They had to deal with whatever element, actions, or attitudes were exacerbating the problem. We could spell out the steps we perceived as necessary for recovery, but the recovery first required forgiveness on their part. The statement of Jesus that a person must first forgive in order to receive God's forgiveness – and a new life – is no mere platitude (Matthew 6:14–15).

So, when other patients saw that one patient had forgiven his domineering father, another a promiscuous mother, or another an overindulgent mother, after years of hating those parents; or when they saw an addict come off heavy doses of heroin and cocaine because of his real love for a woman; or when a son came off heroin because the father he had never known found him after 18 years' search – those patients saw the spiritual values in action, not merely in words.

RE-ENTRY INTO ORDINARY LIFE

We encouraged all our patients to spend at least a week or two, and preferably a month or two, at the end of their 10 days' NET, in some place where they could continue their physical recuperation and become accustomed to the clarity of a mind free of drugs – a painful as well as pleasurable experience, since acuteness of perception was intensified by the restoration of the body's natural production of endorphins. Although our own statistics show no evidence that this helped to prevent recidivism, we still recommend this because of the benefits of better health in dealing with problems.

The most critical stage of recovery is the return to their homes, with all the reminders of their previous habits and the stresses of daily living. Some kind of support system is essential, and the spouse/family of the addict need as much help and guidance as the addict. Actually, the spouse/family should be given as much guidance as possible before the addict leaves the clinic. They, in the presence of the addict, should be warned that it will take time for a relationship of trust to return but that trust will slowly grow as the family see evidence that it is justified.

This can be done with either a verbal understanding between both parties, or a written contract in which a reasonable minimum goal is set to be accomplished, for one week or month or three months. This would include a job to be done, household duties observed, times to get up or go to bed, money to be spent or repaid, etc. When successfully completed, this can be expanded and extended. The family must be strong enough – and love enough – to be able to say 'No' and to stick to that decision no matter what.

Addict and family should also be told if he or she does slip, that, as Stanton Peele says, 'lapses are both understandable and forgivable, and that a lapse should not be a cue to abandon what has been accomplished. In this way, the guilt that is itself a prod to seek the addictive experience is diminished ... people always have a choice, even after they have taken a sip, a puff, or a bite.'[243]

Support systems

Alcoholics Anonymous appears to have helped more alcoholics than any other support system, and Narcotics Anonymous is now trying to fulfil the same function for drug addicts. However, such groups may not be the ideal, because they emphasize negative aspects which keep both alcohol and drugs in the forefront of the addict's mind, instead of replacing them with new positive thoughts and occupations. Also, jealousy of someone else's success very often makes those still addicted want to bring those who are drug-free back down to their own level.

Dr James Ch'ien of Hong Kong, innovator of one of the most active drug rehabilitation programmes in the world, himself reported in 1981: 'In the early years, we found, in spite of the intensity of professional aftercare rendered, the great majority of aftercare clients relapsed to drug use ... The better the aftercare service we provided, the more social dependence that was created.'[55] My personal experience of Dr Ch'ien's work, and other similar programmes, was that the more support systems that were provided during extended rehabilitation, the more dependent the addict became on that system and less able to cope with the pressures of personal and social responsibilities.

Again, Stanton Peele comments:

> The crucial point in judging the benefits of involvement in a group is whether the involvement is an end in itself. If it is, it can be equivalent to the drug or other unhealthy habit it purports to cure. This is the danger of any group which claims that permanent membership in it is the only solution to the problem it is organized to combat ... Membership in a group organized to combat addiction can itself be addictive if it limits participants to one lifestyle, one set of associations, and one way of thinking and feeling.
>
> There is another type of group support that is rarely tried in our society. It involves not the formation of groups on the basis of common addictions, but the use of existing units such as the family

> or work group ... Whether working together on common problems or the problems of one person among them, friends and kin can serve as 'therapists' for one another.[243]

But I must add that only those who have experienced failure as well as strength, forgiveness as well as rejection, love as well as hate, and who are prepared to make *themselves* vulnerable are able to help - and the costs of doing this are as high as the rewards.

During our year in the first NET Clinic in 1980, my husband set up a Befrienders Addiction Counselling Service, and began collecting names of people all over the country who were willing to take one drug addict or alcoholic into their homes, short- or long-term. Those who did so often found the going difficult because of their lack of knowledge and understanding of the nature of addiction, and the monomania which is the central part of the addict's problem.

I was interested to read in a 1984 *Sunday Times* that someone has tried this method with a down-and-out alcoholic - with success. Gary Simcox commented on his experiment six months after the alcoholic had left their home to live in a flat of his own:

> I am disappointed that nobody has come to me to find out how we did it. This was a radical approach, it's not an accepted way of dealing with the problem. A small number of senior people in the caring professions don't like innovation. Professionally what we did is regarded as unacceptable because we got 'too close' to Bernard. The argument is that this will have made him dependent. But that hasn't happened.
>
> The public reaction from all those concerned with helping alcoholics was platitudes. The private one is studied indifference.[96]

We encourage our patients to become actively involved in a specific and, if possible, daily form of exercise, and also in simple stress-reduction techniques. If there is no friend or supportive community or church in their home area to which they can turn, then we recommend sessions at least once weekly with a trained counsellor or clinical psychologist.

Relapse

Quite apart from the results of associating with drug-using friends, craving for the drug or alcohol is likely to return temporarily when any kind of personal crisis occurs. This is where friends and family should do everything possible to alleviate the stress; but if there should be a relapse, nothing should be done to ameliorate the consequences of the relapse - no money given, no rescue from a pub or 'pad', no paying bills or fines - because such actions will 'merely lengthen the time before which (the addict) becomes aware of, and so responsible for, the painful results of his drink (or drug) abuse'.[342]

Relapse can occur in unexpected ways.

> Daniel, very heavily addicted to heroin, methadone and major tranquillizers for many years, showed a dramatic response to NET, changed to a more suitable job when he left the clinic, and experienced no craving at all for over a year. He was then admitted to hospital for a minor operation, given injections of pain-killing drugs before and after the operation - and became re-addicted. Could a skilled anaesthetist not have given an equally effective anaesthetic using only atropine and aspirin? Can doctors not treat the whole patient instead of an isolated condition?

> On the other hand, Jennifer, 23 years old, had been shooting heroin intravenously since she was 15. She went to a sunny island to recuperate after 10 days of NET. When she arrived, every hotel was occupied and she was forced to sleep on the grass in a camping-site. Her craving returned with the difficulties and disappointments. However, the next day she hired a bicycle and, after cycling a few miles, she found a beautiful beach where she could swim and sun-bathe. This enabled her to enjoy her holiday in spite of having to 'camp out' and she had no more craving from that moment.

The joys of being released from the prison of addiction are illustrated by a letter from Johnny, seven years on Valium 100 mg daily and weekend heavy alcoholic bouts, ten months after NET: 'I cannot say how grateful we all are here for my treatment. It unveiled an unknown quality in myself of loving and caring for my family.'

Definition of cure

We are satisfied that rehabilitation is complete when the patient is healed in body, mind and spirit, and has comprehended and shown a capacity to apply a new philosophy of life appropriate to his or her chosen environment.

No longer in bondage to a chemical or behavioural addiction, former addicts can live a life with freedom, joy and love within the family and community. Not many have fully met the above criteria, but 90 per cent are at various stages along the way, with real hope - which is as much as any of us have.

Chapter 10
Spiritual rehabilitation and logotherapy

There is little doubt that the most successful forms of post-detoxification treatment of addictions are those that include a foundational spiritual emphasis in their approach. This may be seen in the work of Alcoholics Anonymous, the Salvation Army, Teen Challenge, and other, non-Christian, organizations. Pamela, who describes her life in the introduction, volunteered the information that not only had *all* her friends become drug addicts, but also that every one of them who had succeeded in remaining drug-free had come to believe in God.

The transforming of the mind

Paul of Tarsus, one of the world's great thinkers and the man most responsible for explaining the true significance of Judaic-Christian philosophy as the revealed mind of God, declared as that philosophy's most fundamental principle:

> Offer your very selves to God; a living sacrifice, dedicated and fit for his acceptance, worship offered by mind and heart. Adapt yourself no longer to the pattern of this present world, *but let your minds be remade and your whole nature thus transformed. Then you will be able to discern the will of God*, and to know what is good, acceptable and perfect. (Romans 12: 1-3, my italics)

There, stated very clearly, are the possibility and the assurance that human nature - even the worst, as Paul affirmed elsewhere - can be transformed by the re-making of the human mind, which learns, in the process, to discern the will of God. At one stroke such a discernment eliminates the problem of emptiness and meaninglessness.

The way to the mind of God by which we may know his will for ourselves is found by making a daily, living sacrifice of our own self-will and allowing the re-making of our own self-centred mind (which by choice and practice has been conditioned to think as 'the natural mind under the spirit of this world') into a similarity to 'the mind of Christ' (Christ was at all times open to the promptings of the Spirit of God regarding his ongoing purposes, and was obedient to them).

The Spirit coming from God prompts our minds, informing us what God desires for us, and evoking in us that desire - the conative impulse - to obey. As we choose to obey or to disobey, the spiritual battle begins, and is resolved as we submit our wills to the choice desired. If the choice is obedience to the mind of God, the Spirit illuminates our minds with an understanding of the commitment, and the same Spirit communicates the decision back to God. This is the process of true prayer.

William Barclay, the noted Scottish theologian, has described this word 'Spirit', or 'Holy Spirit', as 'a word of quite special importance' and 'a word of quite special difficulty'. Almost all translators agree that in many instances it means 'advocate'; but elsewhere it is used to mean 'comforter', 'helper', 'someone who stands with us', or 'he who is to befriend us'. The word itself, *parakletos*, means literally 'one who is called in', and is *passive* in form, but *active in meaning*. The Spirit is always called in to do something, to render some service; to help in some situation with which a person cannot cope.

It is this person in the Judaic-Christian scriptures who delivers us from 'the spirit of bondage to fear', and who brings us in the process of prayer into a new relationship and understanding of a loving heavenly Father. 'The Spirit itself bears witness with our spirit that we are children of God ... the Spirit also helps us in our weakness.'

Because of the presence of the Spirit we are enabled to know and become what we were created to be. Jesus himself submitted to this process when he was 'led by the Spirit into the wilderness' to be tested by the Devil. There Satan used three basic principles, each active in the corruption and destruction of humankind:

(1) *the lust of the flesh* in tempting Jesus to turn stones into bread when hungry - *pleasure* without responsibility;

(2) *the lust of the eyes* in tempting Jesus with material possessions for personal gain - *prestige* without responsibility;

(3) *the pride of life*, tempting Jesus to do miracles for selfish reasons - *power* without responsibility.

These have always been the three basic temptations of humankind, or the three basic drives recognized by psychologists and psychiatrists in Freud's will-to-pleasure, Adler's will-to-power, and Frankl's will-to-meaning. To all of these Jesus found the answer, not in Greek myths, but in scriptural models.

The most difficult step in the transformation process - the long journey from bondage to freedom - is the first: the act of volition, the yielding of the will. The human will includes three aspects of mind: feeling, knowing and conation. We will first take the last mentioned - and least recognized - conation. The conative impulse is the initial desire or aversion which leads to a decision to act. The will comes into play when the person either checks or gives way to the impulse. The essential feature which makes the activity a willed one is that it is the person who decides whether to check the impulse or give it free play. In connection with the theological concept of sin (which means 'a falling short' of God's purpose), it means not only a carrying out of wrong action but a willed consent to wrong action.

Let us return to Paul's words, then, regarding the re-making of the mind through a daily sacrifice of the self. What Paul had in mind was to be God-centred and not self-centred in all the daily decisions of life, to pause between the moment of conation and the moment of choice, and by faith choose what God wants rather than what self wants. In doing this, said Paul, 'through faith ... we are set free'; 'through faith ... we are children of God'.

This is where powerlessness ends and power begins; this is where failure ends and victory begins. This is the critical point in the addicts' experience, the uncrossable hurdle, the unbridgeable gap, which - even after detoxification from the chemical of addiction - has always beaten them and left them without hope, crying out 'I can't', or 'It's impossible.'

Faith in healing

At this point of impossibility, faith, through the Spirit of God, is the cure. Faith, defined by Paul of Tarsus, is 'that which gives substance to our hopes, and makes us certain of realities we do not see'; faith is reaching out for the hand of God - and finding it there. And faith is a gamble; just read Paul's definition once again. It is as good a definition of gambling as can be found; the individual is putting his bet where his hopes are. But faith is also the divinely implanted instinct that enables the believer to grow in the knowledge of God. Gambling, as it has come to be known - placing of money bets for financial profit - is simply the perversion of this faith instinct into material instead of spiritual ends, just as lust is the perversion of love for physical instead of spiritual ends.

Perhaps more than any other thinker, Jung has explored the interrelationship between the physical world and the spiritual world in some 30 volumes, collating evidence from his 80 years to demonstrate that the troublesome emotions of men and women cannot be healed without a radically different view of life and the world, which means taking into full consideration their contacts with the creative centre of meaning.

Jung's psychology is essentially concerned with the search for wholeness, bringing together all the individual's characteristics - good and evil, conscious and unconscious - into the conscious experience of completeness and awareness. He demonstrated that the most advanced thinking supports the conviction that religion is a vitally necessary element in human life, delivering the human spirit from its bondage to a sterile materialism and a meaningless humanism.

Average men and women know little or nothing of this potential intensive or extensive consciousness, little or nothing of the spiritual certainties of their predecessors in earlier centuries (which were characterized by less material obsession and more spiritual provision). Modern ideals of material security, self-centred pursuits, vaguely-defined 'good works', more leisure, pleasure-seeking, and so on, provide no adequate framework for a fulfilled or even mildly satisfying life. Those who turn away from an apparently terrifying prospect of a blind world in which there is increasing chaos, and look inward, find in their own minds even greater chaos and darkness.

But it is just there, in the recesses of the mind that the transformation from chaos to purpose, from darkness to light, from bondage to freedom, must take place. No organic medicine has yet been found to treat neuroses successfully, no proof that psychoneuroses are glandular in nature has been discovered, but psychospiritual methods have been found effective, therapeutic, transforming!

Jung, commenting on the psychic factors effective in curing neuroses, has said:

> For example, a suitable explanation or a comforting word to the patient may have something like a healing effect which may even influence the glandular secretions. The doctor's words, to be sure, are 'only' vibrations in the air, yet they constitute a particular set of vibrations corresponding to a particular psychic state in the doctor. The words are effective only insofar as they convey a meaning or have significance. But meaning is something mental or spiritual. Call it a fiction if you like. None the less it enables us to influence the cause of the disease in a far more effective way than with chemical preparations. We can influence the biochemical processes of the body by it. Whether the fiction arises in me spontaneously, or reaches me from without by way of human speech, it can make me ill or cure me ... Nothing is more effective in the psychic and even psychophysical realm.[161]

Jung, while not a Christian in the orthodox sense, held strong opinions about the phenomenon of evil 'since every psyche is fascinated by it', and he maintained that 'the principal and indeed only thing that is wrong with the world is man'. Further, he held that 'it is only the meaningful that sets us free'.[171]

But for the 'meaning' to make a difference in the individual concerned there has to be understanding of some kind between the speaker and the listener - a state of 'conditional readiness' which activates response. For example, as has been noted, a conversation fundamentally begins when a puff of air, produced by vibrations of the speaker's larynx, echoes around the cavities of the mouth and results in a characteristic sequence of sound waves travelling through space and vibrating the sensitive membranes of the listener's ear, giving rise to nerve impulses, and so on. Where does 'meaning' conveyed and received come into this process? Whether the speaker is a genius elucidating an astounding truth, or an idiot jabbering nonsense, the medium of communication is the same.

How to have a fully equipped mind

The writer of the Book of Hebrews declared that mature individuals were those 'who have their faculties trained by practice to distinguish between good and evil'.

The perception that leads to memory, understanding and will and eventually to wisdom is a faculty that can be trained. However, if it is never used it can atrophy and become a wasted asset, like its physical counterparts.

The Greeks, according to Dr William Barclay, had three important words to describe the three great qualities of mind; any man or woman who had these had 'a mind fully equipped'. They were as follows.

(1) *Sophia*, meaning wisdom, the ultimate knowledge of things human and divine, which is nothing less than the knowledge of God. *Sophia* represents the furthest reach of the human mind.

(2) *Phronesis*, meaning prudence. While *sophia* refers primarily to theoretical concepts, *phronesis* is practical and has to do with a person's life, conduct and action. Aristotle defined *phronesis* as 'truth ... concerned with action in relation to the things that are good for human beings'.

(3) *Sunesis*, meaning understanding, is concerned with judgement, the reaching of a conclusion, a synthesis in the sense of 'putting two and two together'; it is the power to distinguish between two separate courses of action, varying values, differing relationships between people; it refers to the ability to test, to distinguish, to evaluate and to form judgement.

In elaborating on these three great qualities of mind, Dr Barclay comments:

> There is clearly growth in wisdom. Although wisdom is not the discovery of the mind, it cannot be obtained without the strenuous activity of the mind. Real wisdom comes when the Spirit of God reaches down to meet the searching mind, but the mind of man must search before God will come to meet it. Wisdom is not for the mentally lazy, although it is a gift of God.[26]

Wisdom is acquired when the thing known is put to its proper use. Understanding is knowing what is that proper use.

That chemicals should be able to provide essential wisdom and understanding, as Dr Timothy Leary stated during the late 1960s and early 1970s, is ludicrous. Arthur Koestler put it very well:

> It is fundamentally wrong, and naive, to expect that drugs can present the mind with gratis gifts - put into it something which is not already there. Neither mystic insights, nor philosophic wisdom, nor creative power, can be provided by pill or injection. The psychopharmacist cannot *add* to the faculties of the brain - but he can, at best *eliminate* obstructions and blockages which impede their proper use. He cannot aggrandize us - but he can, within limits, normalize us; he cannot put additional circuits within the brain, but he can, again within limits, improve the coordination between existing ones, attenuate conflicts, prevent the blowing of fuses, and ensure a steady power supply. That is all the help we can ask for - but if we were able to attain it, the benefits for mankind would be incalculable.[173]

One of the most intriguing questions being thrown up by the discovery of endorphins is the possible part they play in the behaviour of the 'cult-addict' as well as the 'chemical-addict' and the 'person-addict'. The question is this: Does the person who becomes cult-, object- or person-addicted also diminish the production of natural endorphins required to meet life's challenges and the stresses of pain and emotion; and then, under the new stimulus of another cult, object or person, does the body again respond temporarily - until that new addiction in turn is proved inadequate to the individual's current situation? If so, this theory would go a long way towards explaining why genuine 'spiritual healing' can suddenly and dramatically 'cure' individual and group addiction through *intense belief operating as an electrical stimulus for the manufacture and release of endorphins*, while minor cultic fads are usually successful only for short periods because of their superficial character.

These observations arose out of our increasing involvement with patients from different nations, cultures, religions and backgrounds. Why does Hong Kong, with four million Chinese, have the worst drug addiction problem in the world, while mainland China across the border, with almost one billion Chinese, apparently has none? Why did Chinese Maoism produce no chemical addictions while Soviet Marxism struggles with a monumental alcoholism problem? Why is Buddhist meditation so successful in Thailand, with almost a million heroin addicts (that is, when they can get addicts detoxified enough to meditate)? Why does an authoritarian and ascetic religion like Islam have so many heroin and alcohol addicts in areas such as Indonesia and Iran? Why is it that when the environment is changed - politically, culturally, socially, spiritually - there is a direct and often dramatic effect on what had appeared to be the insoluble problem of addictions? In all the questions, the solutions treated seriously the negative factors of emptiness and meaninglessness and their removal, and the positive factors of vision, values, and some form of adequate and applied belief system for individuals and nations.

The real cure for addiction

The cure for addiction, like the cure for tuberculosis, involves fundamental changes in society. For tuberculosis to be removed as a medical and social scourge, more than medication and surgery were required; a new political and social approach to housing, hygiene and diet was needed as well.

Addiction is also a social disease, though much more complex and pernicious than tuberculosis. After detoxification, the re-structuring of family, community, social, political and ecclesiastical values and patterns are essential. The real cure for addiction requires revolution - spiritual revolution.

A recent authoritative article in the *New England Journal of Medicine* by Dr Armand Nicholi, a Harvard psychiatrist, on the subject of the serious, widespread abuse of mind-altering drugs in the USA, sub-titled 'A modern epidemic', declared:

> What motivates such a vast segment of our society to inhale, ingest, or inject into our bodies this wide assortment of mind-altering substances? When asked this question, those who reported using marijuana daily said that they did so primarily to alter how they felt - to help cope with feelings of stress, anger, depression, frustration, or boredom. College students who used LSD said they took the drug to reduce feelings of loneliness and isolation, to enhance creativity and productiveness, to increase social and sexual effectiveness, and to fill a 'moral and spiritual void'. In essence, people take these drugs to alter or escape from a less than tolerable society, and to meet intense emotional needs ...
>
> In addition, a vast body of research has shown that the absence of a parent through death, divorce or a time-demanding job contributes to many forms of emotional disorder, especially the anger, rebelliousness, low self-esteem, depression, and anti-social behaviour that characterize drug users. Changes in child rearing practices and family stability in the United States, beginning several years before

the drug culture evolved, have shifted child care from parents to other agencies. Cross-cultural studies indicate that American parents spend less time with their children than parents in any other nation in the world except England. The accelerating divorce rate in the United States has closely paralleled the rise in drug use, and over half the children under the age of 18 (approximately 13 million) live in a home with one or both parents missing. Moreover poor academic performance, susceptibility to peer influence, and delinquent behaviour (all characteristic of drug users), as well as suicide and homicide, have been found to be more pronounced among children from homes with one or both parents missing or frequently absent.[222]

The need for spiritual revolution of society is also Alexandr Solzhenitsyn's prophetic message to the West, in a different context. As he argues in his books and broadcasts, spiritual solutions to society's problems, and the discarding of useless materialist substitutes now being promulgated, result from true Christian freedom. This is very different from the unlimited freedom of the Western ideal and the Marxist concept of freedom as acceptance of the yoke of necessity; Christian freedom is *self-restriction* - discipline of the self for the sake of others. In Solzhenitsyn's words:

> Once understood and adopted, this principle diverts us - as individuals, in all forms of association, societies and nations - from *outward* to *inward* development, thereby giving us greater spiritual depth.
>
> The turn toward *inward* development, the triumph of inwardness over outwardness, if it ever happens, will be a great turning point in the history of mankind, comparable to the transition from the Middle Ages to the Renaissance. There will be a complete change not only in the direction of our interest and activities but in the very nature of human beings (a change from spiritual dispersal to spiritual concentration), and a greater change still in the character of human societies. If in some places this is destined to be a revolutionary process, these revolutions will not be like earlier ones - physical, bloody and never beneficial - but will be *moral revolutions*, requiring both courage and sacrifice, though not cruelty - a new phenomenon in human history, of which little is yet known and which as yet no one has prophetically described in clear and precise forms.[292]

While I was researching chemical addictions and electrical stimulation, my husband, George, was pursuing research into these philosophical aspects of the problems of behavioural addictions. The variety of patients that we had, with their own complex background of experiences and forms of treatment, provided a fascinating spectrum for investigation - to them as well as to us. We had patients from Iran and Lebanon, Spain and Italy, Germany and France, Argentina and Brazil, of all classes and creeds, and out of our experience with them we worked out, by trial and error, a system of treatment which could be used for both detoxification and rehabilitation. Strictly speaking our system was only peripherally concerned with what is usually meant by 'rehabilitation'. Our primary concern and emphasis was on 'transformation'.

Rehabilitation is normally associated with restoring individuals to what they were before the onset of illness or a deteriorating physical condition. But our treatment was directed towards transforming individuals whose inadequacies had made them, or had contributed towards their becoming, addicts in the first place; it showed them how to become new men and women.

Here I will repeat an excerpt from the writing of Peter Lawrie, already used in an earlier chapter, in order to refresh the reader's memory as to the uniqueness of the problem of treating addicts of all kinds. The treatment of addiction is unlike the treatment of any other condition, as I have tried to show in preceding chapters. The problem has obscure and complex psycho-spiritual roots embedded deeply in family and social relationships. Consequently, the solution must reach down to those deep roots by radical psycho-spiritual means in much the same way that radical surgery must deeply and cleanly deal with a malignancy.

In *Drugs: Medical, Psychological and Social Facts*, Peter Lawrie has accurately described the therapeutic problem:

> Addicts are notoriously resistant to ordinary psychotherapy. One way of looking at this is to observe that analysis depends on communication, on the patient's acceptance of the therapist as a real human being who can have a real effect on him. But the addict's whole life is organized to remove any dependence on humanity; given his drugs he is self-sufficient, able to generate his own satisfactions and guilts and to live a rich emotional life independent of the outside world. He therefore has no motives for communication when things are going well; when he does present himself for treatment it is often not because he wants to be cured of addiction, but because his addiction is not working as it should. *He is a two-time loser who wants to get back to being a one-time loser, not to take the much more*

> *perilous step to being an unloser.* The ordinary psychiatric patient is like a burr, offering many hooks to the world and the therapist - often too many; the therapist's best strategy is to stand still and let his patient attach himself as he will. But the addict is like a nut: smooth and with a thick armour. The only hook he offers is his need for drugs, and that can be satisfied in a number of ways. *To reach the addict, his shell must be cracked.* We might guess that it would be necessary to counter the coercion of opiates with the coercion of therapy.[181] (my italics)

Mission: to confront and convince

If the goal of the treatment was *transformation*, the starting point was *confrontation.* This was not an artificial process derived from the necessity of 'cracking the nut' of the addict, but a spiritual principle described by Jesus Christ, who taught that self-centred individuals who arrogantly alienate themselves from God and others must be halted and turned round; that the self-will must be recognized, admitted, repented of, rejected, and replaced by the forgiveness and love of God; and that this experience will transform the most depraved individuals and deliver them from their bondage.

Jesus taught that the Spirit's work was to convict of sin, and righteousness, and judgement, to guide our minds into all truth, to proclaim things that are to come, and to reveal the mind of God. 'You shall know the truth,' declared Jesus, 'and the truth shall make you free.'

Thus the basis of 'confrontation therapy' was that counselling required convicting and convincing before the transformation of the mind could take place.

BIBLICAL MODELS

In our comprehensive application, analysis and advice were supplied not on the usual pattern of Greek myths but on Biblical models. For example, in the parable of the Prodigal Son in Luke 15, who spent all his substance on riotous living in a far-away country, the merciful and loving father described by Jesus is presented rather than the self-centred and murderous son of Freud's Oedipus. The psychotherapeutic orientation could be loosely described as Frankl-Jungian in general and Judaic-Christian in particular. That is, it agreed with Jung's statement:

> During the past thirty years people from all over the civilized countries on earth have consulted me ... Among all my patients in the second half of life - that is to say, over thirty-five - there has not been one whose problem in the last resort was not that of finding a religious outlook on life. It is safe to say that every one of them felt ill because he had lost that which the living religions of every age have given to their followers, and none of them has been really healed who did not regain his religious outlook.

And again:

> A psycho-neurosis must be understood as the suffering of a human being who has not discovered what life means for him. All creativeness in the life of the spirit arises from a state of mental suffering.[160]

It was this extra spiritual dimension, primarily in a Judaic–Christian context (although every patient was encouraged in the free choice of a belief system) which we sought to provide.

Logotherapy versus psychoanalysis

Dr Victor E. Frankl, of the United States International University, San Diego, is visiting clinical professor at Stanford University, whose book, *Man's Search for Meaning* - among 27 others - the *American Journal of Psychiatry* has called 'perhaps the most significant thinking since Freud and Adler'.

He pioneered logotherapy, which some writers have called 'the third Viennese School of Psychotherapy'. The Greek word *logos* denotes 'meaning', and logotherapy is based on the concept that striving for meaning in one's life is the primary motivational force in human beings. Hence Frankl speaks of a *will-to-meaning* in contrast to the pleasure principle (or, as he would term it, the will-to-pleasure) on which Freudian psychology is centred, as well as in contrast to the will-to-power stressed by Adlerian psychology.[105] In psychoanalysis, patients must tell their therapist things that are sometimes difficult to tell, but in logotherapy patients must hear things that are sometimes disagreeable to hear.

Dr Frankl has stated emphatically that the psychoanalyst who, in unmasking the motives of a patient, does not stop when he is finally confronted with what is authentic and genuine within the patient's own psyche, 'is really unmasking his own cynical attitude, his own nihilistic tendency to devalue and depreciate that which is human in man'.[104]

Frankl has done more than anyone to investigate and elucidate the problems of twentieth century emptiness and meaninglessness since he faced them at the door of the gas ovens of Auschwitz during World War II. He has classified this 'sense of despair over the lack of meaning in life' as 'noögenic neurosis', a new syndrome of twentieth century society. Noögenic (from the Greek '*noos*', meaning 'mind') neuroses have their origin not in the psychological but rather in the noölogical dimension of human experience, and is caused by 'existential frustration'. This is experienced when man's will-to-meaning is frustrated. Because existence itself is the specifically human mode of being, the striving to find a concrete meaning in personal existence is the *will-to-meaning*, and when this is frustrated it results in noögenic rather than psychogenic neurosis. Having defined it, Dr Frankl has postulated and practised a new method of treatment which he has called 'logotherapy'.

He demonstrates that despair over the meaning of life is a very real neurosis, and, just as sexual frustration may lead to neuroses, the frustration of the will-to-meaning may also lead to neuroses. However, noögenic neuroses do not emerge from conflicts between drives and instincts, but rather from conflicts between various values, in other words, from moral conflicts or spiritual problems.

Logotherapy, therefore, aims at breaking up the typical self-centredness of the neurotic – or, as we are discussing from our experience, the addict – instead of continually fostering and reinforcing it, as is the usual practice. It focuses on assignments and meanings to be fulfilled by the patient in his future. It considers the individual as a being whose main concern consists of fulfilling a meaning and in actualizing values, rather than in mere gratification of instincts, mere adaptation and adjustment to society and personal environment. Men and women, in contrast to lesser animals, must have a goal in life.

Frankl asserts:

> A goal can be a goal in life, however, only if it has meaning. Now I am prepared for the argument that psychotherapy belongs to the realm of science and is not concerned with values; but I believe there is no such thing as psychotherapy unconcerned with values, only one that is blind to values. A psychotherapy which not only recognises man's spirit, but actually starts from it, may be termed logotherapy. In this connection, *logos* is intended to signify 'the spiritual'

> and beyond that 'the meaning'. (It must be kept in mind, however, that within the framework of logotherapy 'spiritual' does not have a religious connotation but refers to the specifically human dimension.)[104]

Frankl points out that it is not the aim of logotherapy to take the place of existing psychotherapy, but only to complement it, thereby forming a picture of men and women in their wholeness, which must include the spiritual dimension. Psychotherapy, he argues, as it has been developed up until the present, needs to be supplemented by a procedure which operates beyond the field of the Oedipus complex and the inferiority complex, or, in more general terms, beyond all affect-dynamics. 'What is still missing,' he declares, 'is a form of psychotherapy which gets underneath psychodynamics, which sees beneath the psychic malaise of the neurotic, his spiritual struggles ... What we are concerned with is a psychotherapy in spiritual terms.'[104]

SUPERFICIAL RELIGIOUS FORMULAE

Noted theologian Paul Tillich has defined *emptiness* and *meaninglessness* as the two levels of a threatening experience of non-being which attack spiritual affirmation, emptiness being the relative threat, and meaninglessness being the absolute threat. The anxiety of meaninglessness is 'anxiety about the loss of an ultimate concern of a meaning which gives meaning to all meaning'. This anxiety is aroused by the loss of a spiritual centre or locus and by a conscious lack of knowledge of the meaning of existence. This loss of spiritual centre, which leads to a loss of the meaning of life, Tillich maintains, follows the loss of God in the lives of individuals:

> The decisive event which underlies the search for meaning and despair of it in the twentieth century is the loss of God in the nineteenth century. Feuerbach explained God away in terms of the infinite desire of the human heart; Marx explained him away in terms of an ideological attempt to rise above the given reality; Nietzsche as a weakening of the will to live. The result is the pronouncement; 'God is dead,' and with him the whole system in which one lived.[312]

Ever since the institutional churches opted out of their social and political responsibilities in the seventeenth century, followed by the end of ecclesiastical paternalism in the nineteenth century, Western society has lost its 'spiritual centre' and has found no spiritual corpus to replace it. In the past 20 years alone, Britain has imported nearly 100 so-called religions – mainly from America, India, and the Far East – and, according to one newspaper report, 'some are entirely innocent, some are fads, some are confidence tricks, some are products of eccentrics; a few are sinister'. To paraphrase G. K. Chesterton: When a person or nation gives up belief in God they do not believe in no gods but in any gods.

For where there is no chemical addiction – and often where there is – there is behavioural addiction in an attempt to fill the emptiness and meaninglessness in the individual and society. There is the ludicrous but sinister Unification Church of South Korea, better known as the Moonies. There was the crypto-Communist People's Temple of megalomaniac Jim Jones, which posed as a Christian organization to tap the moneyed sources of jaded Christianity in America while extorting money from its poor members in order to set up a Marxist commune in Guyana, with the whole affair ending in a holocaust of suicide and notoriety.

There was the subtle and intimidating drug-rehabilitation organization of Synanon, founded by ex-alcoholic Charles Dederich, with no known 'spiritual centre' but with 'the Game', an empirical individualist philosophy in which members denounced each other in order to work off their hostilities and gain meaningful relationships. There are the Children of God, with their notorious reputation of sexual enticement as 'hookers for Jesus' while insisting that they are the only true believers. There are the many bizarre Eastern cultic imports – Transcendental Meditation, Divine Light Mission, the sex-oriented Bhagwan Shree Rajneesh movement and the extremist Ananda Marg. There is also, of course, the Christian Pentecostal movement, actively propagating their arbitrary selection of some six 'charismatic gifts', out of a Biblical availability of about 30, and sometimes being just as cultic by definition and exclusivity as their more notorious counterparts.

Implicit in all of this ritualized obsession is a critical lack of values elsewhere in modern society – that same sickness lying at the root of the problem of addicts noted by the Council of Europe in its report (see pages 52–55) – and a widespread hunger and search for values and meaning. The great deceit at the heart of the problem, however, perpetuated by twentieth century doctors, is that chemicals with power to produce an altered state of consciousness, or behavioural addictions with a similar result, are an adequate substitute for the real thing. Addicts know that they are being conned, and only despair drives them from one to another as a last resort.

It is evident that in the future doctors will have to emphasize spiritual meaning and well-being as well as the medical in the treatment of sickness. This is especially true in the treatment of conditions associated with the mind, such as addictions.

In using logotherapy Frankl emphasized that the logotherapist is neither a teacher nor preacher. If he or she has a personal belief system it is for that individual alone and for the interested individual who asks about it. Changing the metaphor, the logotherapist is not a painter, but an eye specialist. A painter paints the world as he or she sees it; the eye specialist enables the individual to see the world as it is.

The world as it is is not merely an expression of one's self; nor is it a vehicle or instrument to give one's self significance or meaning. The world is the place, or the combination of circumstances and experiences, within which one aspect of human existence and meaning is to be found; the other aspect is found within men and women who live in that world, in their own psyche.

That is why so-called 'self-actualization' will never succeed in providing satisfaction or meaning; it is only half the solution. The full solution lies in self-transcendence, of which self-actualization is but the side-effect. Like sex without love, self-actualization without self-transcendence leads to satiety and not to satisfaction.

THREE PATHS TO MEANING

According to logotherapy, therefore, the meaning of life can be discovered in three different ways: one, by doing a deed; two, by experiencing a value; three, by suffering. The first is found in *the accomplishment of a set task*, the second by *experiencing truth* - beauty, mercy, justice, right-doing (for example, in loving a person - lover, spouse, or neighbour - as one's self). The third way to find meaning is by *suffering*; by seeking and finding the lesson in some trial or crisis experience; understanding, absorbing and profiting from it; working through it, sharing it with others and growing because of it.

A profound and challenging example of this was Dr Frankl's own experience in facing the ultimate horror in the twentieth century - the gas chamber holocaust of Auschwitz:

> Let me recall that which was perhaps the deepest experience I had

in the concentration camp. The odds of surviving the camp were no more than one to twenty-eight, as can be verified by exact statistics. It did not even seem possible, let alone probable, that the manuscript of my first book, which I had hidden in my coat when I arrived at Auschwitz, would ever be rescued. Thus, I had to undergo and to overcome the loss of my spiritual child. And now it seemed as if nothing and no one would survive me; neither a physical nor a spiritual child of my own! So I found myself confronted with the question of whether under such circumstances my life was ultimately void of any meaning.

Not yet did I notice that an answer to this question with which I was wrestling so passionately was already in store for me, and that soon thereafter this answer would be given to me. This was the case when I had to surrender my clothes and in turn inherited the worn-out rags of an inmate who had been sent to the gas chamber immediately after his arrival at the Auschwitz railway station. Instead of the many pages of my manuscript, I found in the pocket of the newly acquired coat a single page torn out of a Hebrew prayer book, which contained the main Jewish prayer, *Shema Yisrael.* How should I have interpreted such a 'coincidence' other then as a challenge to *live* my thoughts instead of merely putting them on paper?

A bit later, I remember, it seemed to me that I would die in the near future. In this critical situation, however, my concern was different from that of most of my comrades. Their question was, 'Will we survive the camp? For, if not, all this suffering has no meaning.' The question which beset me was, 'Has all this suffering, this dying around us, a meaning? For, if not, then ultimately there is no meaning to survival; for a life whose meaning depends on such a happenstance - whether one escapes or not - ultimately would not be worth living at all.'[104]

It is interesting to reflect further on the use of the term *logos* in bringing back an individual to a spiritual centre. The concept of the *logos* in the Judaic-Christian and Greek classical sense has played a profound part in the development of Western civilization, but there is also a significant parallel in the recent transformation of Chinese society through Chairman Mao Zedong's definition of the generic Chinese word *szuh-siang*, meaning 'correct thinking'.[235]

Logos, as Frankl says, is a Greek word, but the concept behind it is rooted in Judaic-Greek etymology. To the Jews, *logos*, 'the word', was not merely a sound but a dynamic force, the *Word* of God by which he created the world, the very idea of the action of God, the creative and illuminating power of God, enabling the object of its interest to accomplish his purpose. To the Greeks, *logos* was the *reason* of God, the principle of order under which the universe continued to exist; a purpose, a plan, a design, the mind of God controlling the world and every man and woman in it. It was the combination of these two streams of thought that gave to the Apostle John his conception of Jesus Christ as 'the Word of God made flesh' – the unique revelation of Christianity.

SIGNIFICANCE OF MAOISM

But, taking up Frankl's point that logotherapy – as he uses the term and technique – is not necessarily religious, but is integrally related to the human dimension and aspiration, as indicated above, it is fascinating to study the similar technique developed and practised in China by the late Chairman Mao. His uniquely personal form of 'spiritual' Marxism was used to transform a nation of some 800 million inhabitants, disillusioned and despairing over the lack of meaning in their lives, to forge them into a new people with vision, values and meaning. In order to create such a 'new society', with 'new men' and 'new women', he had to create a new form of revolution – which he did through what is now known worldwide as 'Maoism'.

While Western intellectuals nibbled peripherally at the problems confronting a dying Western society and their possible solutions, falling back defeated into reductionism and nihilism, Chairman Mao was switching his almost one-billion (one-third of the world) nation from being one of the world's most drug-addicted, despairing, and defeated societies to being the greatest cult-addicted but vital society by means of a psychospiritual process. Earlier Hitler had achieved something similar with Nazism, his hybrid amalgam of vision, values and meaning in National Socialism, which transformed Germany. Obviously, these were perversions of a process inherent in humankind and society which could be harnessed to higher goals.

In the first two decades of the twentieth century in China, doubt and uncertainty – the twin constituent elements in the condition of anxiety – had replaced the traditional pride and confidence. Chinese intellectuals then turned to the West in search of its apparently successful ideas, and discovered the materialist Marxism, so alien to its history and traditions. Like personal doubts and uncertainties, group or national doubts and uncertainties regarding the viability of social structures, once they are successfully challenged, operate in similar fashion in that they empty the system of existing values and ideas, leaving hopelessness, disillusion, and despair. When it is seen that the previous ideas and values no longer accurately articulate the human situation, they become increasingly destructive and are powerless to solve the human situation. (In the West in this century, this is evident in the collapse of the ecclesiastical symbols of Christianity, the political symbols of democracy, and the ideological symbols of Marxism.)

China had tried institutionalized democracy and ecclesiastical Christianity. Both had failed because they were already failing in the West. But Marxism was still relatively new in the early 1920s, and the debate in China centred around whether Marxism's developing institutional form in Soviet Russia was applicable to China, or whether its earlier dynamic ideas and values as articulated by the young Marx and adapted to China were more relevant. China's intellectuals chose the latter, which evolved into Maoism.

The Maoist vision was both particular and universal. Particular in that the People's Republic of China was seen as the spiritual centre and source of inspiration and the example for people's liberation movements everywhere; universal in that it postulated a giant moral battle on a global scale between the forces of good and the forces of evil, while that same moral struggle took place in the life of each individual. It was also intensely evangelistic and, as a consequence, became messianic and eschatological, deifying Mao in the present and envisioning a new, utopian age through Maoist principles of world revolution.

The transformation of men and women, from being 'self-centred' to being 'others-centred' was fundamental to the success of the whole revolution, and in this conception and campaign Mao not only matched the young idealist Marx, but surpassed him and other Marxist leaders.

Self-interest was the original sin of the Maoist spiritual concepts. In study sessions throughout the country all students and teachers had to practice 'self-criticism', confess 'self-interest', and 'thoroughly destroy self-interest' in order to uphold the concept of 'teaching for revolution and learning for revolution'. It was self-interest, Mao said, which produced careerism, individualism, elitism, avarice, profiteering, pursuit of fame, and privilege. Within a few years the majority of Chinese were convinced that salvation through 'struggle-criticism-transformation' was readily, if laboriously, possible, because they had seen the conversion process work. Mao's 'Thought' was said to generate *szu-hsiang*, meaning 'correct thought', and this was the determinant of all action, 'translating doctrine into reality, and sustaining people's faith in the darkest hour'.

Despite its dramatic impact, it was evident that Maoism was inadequate to meet China's needs; its demonstrable weakness confirmed the axiom that 'a spiritual centre', or spiritual corpus, cannot be produced at will simply to support a political or cultural system; it has to be the mainspring, the inspiration, of such a system, rising from the people upwards and descending from the authorities downwards. Without such an inspirational spiritual centre, or corpus, there is an inevitable separation, a lack of integration, from the whole of reality, an isolation of the individual self, a sense of non-identity with or non-participation in cosmic or divine purpose.

The dissatisfied individuals then tend to break away from the less concerned mass and form smaller, then larger, groups in order to identify themselves with something supra- or trans-individual. This helps to alleviate their sense of alienation, emptiness and meaninglessness by accepting another imposed authority in place of the weak or inadequate father, or parents, or government, or church; surrendering their freedom to question, finding solutions for their immediate problems in uncritically accepting strongly affirmed answers to vaguely postulated and usually specious questions. In order to allay the increasing pangs of anxiety brought on by the increasing emptiness and meaninglessness as they move from one idiosyncratic group to another, these individuals or groups eventually retreat from challenging freedom to a robotomorphic situation which discourages disturbing questions and encourages packaged answers.

The new framework

To return to our clinic, our counselling was based on the conviction that life held an ultimate meaning and that this was knowable by any individual who was prepared to seek it out. The goal of the treatment was to provide the individual with a compass with which to begin a new journey, and to let him or her experience the excitement of discovering a new world of which he or she was a meaningful part. In the words of poet Christopher Fry:

Thank God our time is now, when wrong
Comes up to meet us everywhere
Never to leave us till we take
The longest stride of soul man ever took –
Affairs are now soul size
The enterprise
Is exploration into God.

Patients were encouraged to look at their chosen environment from a different viewpoint, with a different set of values, which would instil meaning instead of despair, enabling them to break out of the prison of self-interest, the monomania of 'me first' and 'me only', which had brought them to where they were. Our goal was to provide them with a framework of knowledge 'adequate to the thing to be known', or, more precisely, adequate to their chosen environment (for which they were responsible) in order to cure the underlying emptiness and meaninglessness resulting from a previous lack of adequate values.

Obviously, in the short time spent at the clinic it was not possible to provide a complete philosophy of life for every patient. But keeping in mind that our goal was only to give patients a compass, let me give an example of our approach.

Imagine a person who has a fear of water, and cannot swim. To give him a philosophy to explain fear, or an explanation of Archimedes' principle, or the formula for the constituent elements of water, or all of these plus a theology of God as Creator, would be useless. Instead, you must teach him how to dog paddle by getting into the water with him, supporting his chin, getting his hands and legs moving, then standing back as he begins to swim on his own. At that point the fear goes, and enjoyment starts – and he becomes receptive to this new mode of progress. Next, he wants to swim the length of the pool, then to learn the crawl and backstroke. He is eager to sail a boat, a yacht, and to venture out on the ocean instead of being content with quiet harbour sailing. He learns about currents and winds and stars. He has accepted a new philosophy of life – and all because he learned to dog paddle.

In the time at the clinic, therefore, the aim was to uncover the patients' basic problems, find solutions based on values related to a philosophy of life and, when the patients saw it working, launch them with confidence and even enjoyment in the world that had formerly defeated them. It had worked for us; why should it not work for them? Was their basic problem bitterness against a father, or mother, or wife, or husband? Then get the parent or spouse to come to the clinic, discuss the problem separately, then together, and get both parties to begin to practise love and forgiveness instead of hate and resentment. There is nothing so healing to the spirit as forgiveness. Try it for a week or a month. Try it with a written contract or a verbal agreement, if necessary, to overcome doubt and scepticism. But *try* it. Don't just theorize. *Act* on the basis of those values, expressing responses of love instead of responses of hate, practising forgiveness, when there were lapses, instead of recrimination and resentment. And it worked.

THE SPIRITUAL ELEMENT

The cure of addiction requires not only a spiritual point of departure - an assumption that the spiritual is an essential part of human nature - but also a spiritual centre around which all activity revolves, and a spiritual goal towards which the individual progresses. It is this spiritual orientation which gives meaning to life.

Logotherapy ultimately educates a person towards accepting responsibility. Blind response to a stimulus is what happens to animals - *vide* Pavlov's salivating dogs - but acceptance of responsibility can only be undertaken properly by those who understand the implications of the response stimulus. The addict is a confident and experienced liar whose obsession with self-indulgence has forced him to lie to parents, to spouse, to children, to employer, to police, to doctor, to pharmacists, to fellow addicts, to family, to friends, to relatives, in a widening web of deceit that feeds on the measure of its success. This has been described by one experienced writer:

> His (the addict's) conception of himself is that of a fairly worthless creature who can hardly move about in society without a constant barrage of anxiety. (With drugs) he leaves the world of symbolic interaction behind in one fundamental sense; for although he may continue to function as a medical practitioner, a musician, etc., he is no longer dependent on it for his sense of self-value.[132]

Our treatment was built around Frankl's *four basic symptoms*, and Jung's *four basic faculties*. Frankl defines collective neurosis as comprising four basic symptoms:

(1) a planless, goalless, day-to-day attitude towards life;

(2) a fatalistic attitude towards life;
(3) collective thinking, or abandonment of free and responsible decisions; and
(4) fanaticism, or blind following of self-opinion. (It was the Spanish philosopher George Santayana who said: 'Fanaticism consists of redoubling your effort when you have forgotten your aim.') All of these lead to 'the pathological spirit of our time as a mental epidemic'. These four symptoms are characteristically recognizable to anyone who works with drug addicts and alcoholics.

But, Frankl continues, as long as man is capable of conflict of conscience he will be immune to fanaticism and to collective neuroses in general. Conversely, one who suffers from collective neurosis will overcome it if he or she is enabled once more to hear the voice of conscience, and suffer from it: 'Ultimately, all of these four symptoms can be traced back to man's fear of responsibility and his escape from freedom. Yet responsibility and freedom comprise the spiritual domain of man.'[104]

Carl Jung saw human beings as possessing four basic faculties: sensation, thinking, feeling and intuition. Some people have more of one than another, but everyone needs a balance of all four 'faculties' to be a healthy human being. The four faculties correspond to the obvious means by which consciousness obtains its orientation to experience.

Jung went on to define the four faculties: *sensation* (or sense perception) which tells us that something exists; *thinking*, which tells us what it is; *feeling*, which tells us whether it is agreeable or not; and *intuition*, which tells us where it comes from and where it is going. When those four basic faculties are not in proper balance, 'disorders' occur, thrusting the individual into doubt and uncertainty, the twin pillars that reinforce anxiety, stress and drug abuse.

Returning to Frankl, who believed that 'being human means being conscious and being responsible', we also note the characteristics of healthy human existence he specified: (1) education in responsibility; (2) education in freedom to decide; and (3) education in spirituality. These three characteristics are necessary to combat emptiness and meaninglessness.

The gap between the three factors which characterize healthy human existence and the four basic symptoms of despair over meaninglessness is the gap which must be bridged through the four faculties listed by Jung, as illustrated in Figure 10.1.

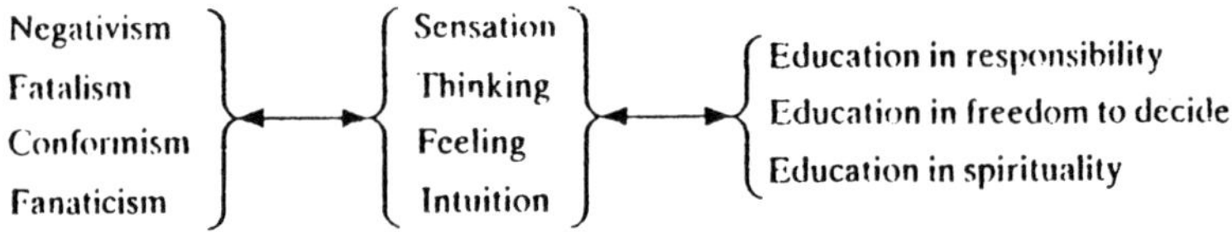

Figure 10.1

TRUE FREEDOM WITH RESPONSIBILITY – THE GOAL

The purpose of our treatment process is to help patients understand the meaning of freedom and responsibility and apply them in life. Frankl states that 'in the end, education must be education towards the ability to decide', and that what is presented for decision must not only be a comprehensive and relative 'framework of meaning', but also leave the individual with the knowledge of ultimate responsibility and freedom to choose acceptance or rejection.

Freedom is a relative term in any language, philosophy or religion. Jean Jacques Rousseau declared: 'Man is born free, but he is everywhere in chains.' Socrates said: 'How can you call a man free when his pleasures rule over him?' We quote again what Solzhenitsyn has written in our own day:

> Save through self-restriction there is no other true freedom for mankind. After the Western ideal of unlimited freedom, after the Marxist concept of freedom as acceptance of the yoke of necessity – here is the true Christian concept of freedom. Freedom is *self-restriction*! Restriction of the self for the sake of others!
>
> Once understood and adapted, this principle diverts us – as individuals, in all forms of human associations, societies and nations – from *outward* to *inward* development, thereby giving us greater spiritual depth.[292]

Solzhenitsyn's definition of freedom parallels that of India's sage-philosopher-poet, Rabindrinath Tagore, who wrote: 'Freedom from the bondage of the soil is no liberty for the tree.'

It is this concept of freedom that has its unique origins in the Judaic-Christian scriptures which have moulded so many of Western civilization's ideals. It involves freely forsaking the bondage to self, and willingly accepting the bondage to God. As Bob Dylan sings, 'You gotta serve somebody.'

RECOGNIZING TRUTH

Regarding the significant place of truth in deliverance from self-bondage, it is worth repeating once more what Jesus declared: 'If you continue in my words, then are you my disciples indeed: and you shall know the truth, and the truth shall make you free.'

Jesus was not just declaring a principle of universal value, important as that would be (for the observance of a recognized standard of truth in personal, group, national, and international relationships would set individuals, communities, and nations free from the bondage and consequences of lying, hypocrisy and deceit). But he was categorically asserting that it is possible for an individual to know the truth, as a divine absolute which Jesus himself had received from God his Father. As a result, that individual would be delivered from all the consequences of experienced bondage.

But, like jesting Pilate, it may be asked: 'What is truth?' Archbishop William Temple gives this working definition: 'Truth is the objective apprehension of things as they are, in contrast to an apprehension or vision distorted by selfish desires and special interests.'[308]

A restatement of the meaning of freedom, therefore, as Jesus taught it, would be: '*Freedom* is knowing the general and particular *truth* revealed by God the Father regarding his purpose in creation, and in perceiving and practising that revealed truth.'

In Archbishop Temple's words again, this would read: 'The way to spiritual freedom ... is always by surrender to the object - to the real facts in the life of science, to the goal or cause in practical conduct, to God as he reveals himself in worship.'

At the clinic we taught that, to remain free from drugs, an individual has to become God-centred instead of self-centred, God-controlled instead of self-directed. For it is self-interest which is the bondage of the addict. He or she is not just in bondage to a chemical, as has been demonstrated by detoxification from its effects; the true bondage is the addiction to a life-style of impotence - even at the price of its accompanying self-loathing. It is not just the drug-free life which is without meaning; it is the inner self which is devoid of values.

BELIEF AND VALUES

A person has to have a belief if he or she is to have values - a belief that is more than a mere mental assent to a set of propositions. A value may be defined as a belief freely chosen from among alternatives after careful consideration of the consequences of each alternative; a belief that is prized, so that the person is happy with the choice; a belief that is important enough that the person will publicly affirm the choice; a belief that is acted on repeatedly, over a period of time, and incorporated into a person's behaviour.

To provide patients with the opportunity to find such a belief system, we emphasized three groups of values.

(1) *Creative values* were inculcated by achieving specific tasks, starting with meditation and other exercises to provide a framework within which to experience a wider and deeper spiritual appreciation of life. Physical and emotional re-education by means of various techniques for living were used to teach self-discipline as a start.

(2) *Experiential values* were discovered by putting into practice fundamental principles learned at study or interaction groups during discussions of practical religion and philosophy, about what is right, good, true, beautiful, pure, just, etc. Involvement in a community where the lessons learned could be tested and proved was found to be essential.

(3) *Personal values* included the correcting of 'personality disorders' by spiritual means. Caring counsellors provided the individual with a sense of security, self-reliance, and self-confidence. The goal was to help the individual grasp the possibility of being a significant person with a meaningful role to play in the family and community. That sense of meaning was acquired by each individual in a framework of loving and being loved in a unique, specific, and personal way. The individuals who had come that far were encouraged to communicate their new sense of meaning to at least one other person so that he or she could share that uniqueness.

A FAMILY MODEL

What this meant for us as a family was that my relations with my husband and ours with our children, were under constant daily scrutiny by every addict. We ate, lived, worked with them on the principle that patients were to be treated as we treated each other. We did not ask them to do what we were not doing ourselves. If the results were good for us and our children, and the addicts liked what they saw, then it was likely to be good for them. That was what 'loving your neighbour as yourselves' meant to us. We loved each other's company, and we were glad to share what we had as a family and as professionals with some experience of the addicts' problems; but that was because our lives were founded on spiritual values acquired in difficult experiences in several countries and cultures.

Professor Einstein of Jerusalem, Editor of the *International Journal of the Addictions*, wrote in a 1984 editorial entitled, 'Coping and drug misuse intervention':

> Many of us may not know how to go beyond the concept of coping in our own lives. In order that we can help others who are stigmatized, maladaptive copers, we would be forced to *join with them* in a mutual venture, rather than continue to treat them as we currently do at a *therapeutic distance.*[99] (Einstein's italics)

The concept of a clinic using treatment in which doctors, nurses, counsellors and patients are mutually and constructively involved in the treatment process has been demonstrated very successfully in California in the United States. The clinic gained nationwide and then worldwide publicity when the former US President, Gerald Ford's wife, Betty, went there for treatment of her addiction to alcohol and drugs, and then spoke out in its favour afterwards. Since that time she has set up her own Betty Ford Center, based on the same procedures, for the treatment of addictions of all kinds, and a stream of famous personalities - Elizabeth Taylor, Liza Minnelli, Robert Mitchum, Tony Curtis among them - have now been treated successfully there.

The emphasis is on 'honesty, courage, and love', but 'most of all, humility', because, according to Betty Ford, of the need to 'recognize that only a power greater than you can lead you to sanity'.

There are no private rooms at the clinic and everybody, no matter how eminent, has at least one person sharing the room. Every person is expected to make his or her own bed, wash up, sweep, take out the rubbish, without exception. 'My first job was to take the garbage out, and hose down the patio', Elizabeth Taylor has said. 'I was very proud of the patio. As for the garbage - well, it's something that has to be done. You do it, and you don't even think about it, and everybody else is doing their own thing.'

The doing of these apparently trivial but necessary everyday domestic tasks, the attitude of individuals towards doing them, and the manner of doing them, are all important aspects of psycho-spiritual therapy and part of the healing process.

The family of the addict is not only requested but *required* to attend the Betty Ford Center, for lectures and therapy to help understand the problem of addiction. The patients have a compulsory reading list of books from Alcoholics Anonymous, including those emphasizing spiritual values. Addicts in the clinic are forced to look rationally and honestly at themselves, and at their actions, guided by caring and compassionate counsellors; and it is not uncommon to find famous people weeping uncontrollably for the first time in many years as they confront their real motivations. This is often distressing, they admit, but it forces them to reassess values and priorities, and often revolutionizes their lives.

Elizabeth Taylor said: 'Everyone tells you they love you, but (in the clinic) they have to name specific things that you have done that caused them pain, anger, humiliation, and so on.'

The ultimate aim

To describe such a clinic and treatment process for addiction, like our own in Britain, is to demonstrate how unique and radical public, professional and official attitudes will have to be if the problem of addiction is ever to be solved. What is involved is a healing of body, mind and spirit; a transformation of personal and social relationships; a practicable integration of the scientific and the psycho-spiritual to meet the challenges of detoxification and rehabilitation; and a realistic awareness of the scale of political/economic issues directly and indirectly related.

The aim of the doctor at all times must be to bring out the greatest potential of the patient, to realize his or her latent values. Goethe said: 'If we take people as they are, we make them worse. If we treat them as if they were what they ought to be, we help them to become what they are capable of becoming.' In this context, Dr Frankl said: 'To experience one human being as unique means to love him.' And Dostoevsky summed it all up when he said: 'To love a person means to see him as God intended him to be.'

Appendix I
References

1 Acupuncture Anaesthesia. Peking: Foreign Languages Press, 1973.

2 Adam K, Adamson L, Brezinova V, Hunter WM. Nitrazepam: lastingly effective but trouble on withdrawal. Br Med J 1976;1:1558-60.

3 Adams JE. Naloxone reversal of analgesia produced by brain stimulation in the human. Pain 1976;2:161-6.

4 Akil H, Liebeskind JC. Monoaminergic mechanisms of stimulation-produced analgesia. Brain Res 1975;94:279-96.

5 Akil H, Mayer DJ. Antagonism of stimulation-produced analgesia by p-CPA, a serotonin synthesis inhibitor. Brain Res 1972;44:692-70.

6 Akil H, Mayer DJ, Liebeskind JC. Antagonism of stimulation-produced analgesia by naloxone, a narcotic antagonist. Science 1976;191:961-2.

7 Akil H, Richardson DE, Hughes J, Barchas JD. Enkephalin-like material elevated in ventricular cerebrospinal fluid of pain patients after analgetic focal stimulation. Science 1978;201:463-5.

8 Alcohol problem of women and young people. National Council of Women 1976.

9 Alexander P, Hamilton Fairley G, Smithers DW. Repeated acupuncture and serum hepatitis. Br Med J 1974;2:466.

10 Altura BT, Altura BM. Phencyclidine, lysergic acid diethylamide and mescaline: cerebral artery spasms and hallucinogenic activity. Science 1981;212:1051-2.

11 Andersen K. Crashing on cocaine. Time 1983 April 11:22-31.

12 Anokhina IP, Brusov OS, Nechaev NV, Balashov AM, Beliaev NA, Panchenko LF. Effect of acute and chronic ethanol exposure on the rat brain opiate receptor function. Alcohol and Alcoholism 1983;18:21-6.

13 Anonymous. An absence of alcohol policy (Editorial). Br Med J 1982;285:1680-1.

14 Anonymous. Clonidine and methyldopa - any role for hypertension now? Drug and Therapeutics Bulletin 1984;22:42.

15 Anonymous. Clonidine for opiate withdrawal (Editorial comment). Lancet 1980;ii:649.

16 Anonymous. Electrical stimulation of the brain (Editorial). Lancet 1974;ii:562-4.

17 Anonymous. How does acupuncture work? (Editorial). Lancet 1981;ii:746-8.

18 Anonymous. New moves on smoking. Br Med J 1985;290:865.

19 Anonymous. Opiates, opioid peptides, and immunity (Editorial). Lancet 1984;i:774-5.

20 Asberg M, Traskman L, Thoren P. 5-HIAA in the cerebrospinal fluid. Arch Gen Psychiatry 1976;33:1193.

21 Ashton H. Benzodiazepine withdrawal: an unfinished story. Br Med J 1984;288:1135-40.

22 Ausubel DP. Methadone maintenance treatment: the other side of the coin. International J Addictions 1983;18:851-62.

23 Badawy AA, Evans M. Opposite effects of chronic administration and subsequent withdrawal of drugs of dependence on the metabolism and disposition of endogenous and exogenous tryptophan in the rat. Alcohol and Alcoholism 1983;18:369-82.

24 Banks A, Waller TAN. Drug Addiction and Polydrug Abuse: The role of the General Practitioner. London: Library and Information Service for the Study of Drug Dependence, 1983.

25 Banshchikov VM, Sudakov HV, Kulikova YI, Arsentyev DA. Behavioural and electroencephalographic responses in a state of electrically induced sleep. In: Wageneder FM, Germann RH, eds. Electrotherapeutic Sleep and Electroanaesthesia. Vol III. Third International Symposium in Varna. Graz: RM Verlag, 1974.

26 Barclay William. New Testament Words. Philadelphia: The Westminster Press, 1976.

27 Becker RO. Electromagnetic forces and life processes. Technology Rev 1972;75:2-8.

28 Becker RO. The basic biological data transmission and control system influenced by electrical forces. Ann NY Acad Sci 1974;238:236-41.

29 Becker RO, Marino AA. Electromagnetism and Life. Albany: State University of New York Press, 1982:14-7.

30 Ben-Sreti MM, Gonzalez JP, Sewell RDE. The influence of selective dopaminergic and cholinergic agonists and antagonists on precipitated opiate abstinence. Alcohol and Alcoholism 1983;18:353-9.

31 Berdyaev Nicolas. Freedom and The Spirit, 1935. New York: Irvington, 1982.

32 Beswick FB, Conroy RTWL. Optimal tetanic conditioning of heteronymous monosynaptic reflexes. J Physiol 1965;180:134-46.

33 Bloom F, Bayon A, Battenberg E, et al. Endorphins: developmental, cellular and behavioral aspects. In: Costa E, Trabucchi M, eds. Neural Peptides and Neuronal Communication. New York: Raven Press, 1980:619-32.

34 Bloom F, Segal D, Ling N, Guillemin R. Endorphins: profound behavioral effects in rats suggest new etiological factors in mental illness. Science 1976;194:630-2.

35 Blum K. Handbook of Abusable Drugs. New York and London: Gardner Press Inc, 1984:47,696,701.

36 Borg S, Kvande H, Mossberg D, Sedvall G. Central nervous noradrenaline metabolism in alcoholics during long-term abstinence. Alcohol and Alcoholism 1983;18:321-3.

37 Borgens RB, Roederer E, Cohen MJ. Enhanced spinal cord regeneration in lamprey by applied electrical fields. Science 1981;213:611-7.

38 Braestrup C, Nielsen M, Olsen CE. Urinary and brain β-carboline-3-carboxylates as potent inhibitors of brain benzodiazepine receptors. Proc Natl Acad Sci 1980;77:2288-92.

39 Brecher EM. Licit and Illicit Drugs. Boston: Little, Brown and Company, 1972:64.

40 Brewer Colin. World Medicine 1977 May 18.

41 Brook MG. Psychosis after cannabis abuse. Br Med J 1984;288:1381.

42 Brown LB, Goodwin FK, Ballenger JC, Goyer PF, Major LF. Aggression in humans correlates with cerebrospinal fluid amine metabolites. Psychiatry Research 1979;1:131-9.

43 Brown NM, Strachen JW. Analgesia in acute pancreatitis. Br Med J 1984;288:1917.

44 Burroughs W. Junkie. London: New English Library, 1969:11.

45 Capel ID, Goode IG, Patterson MA. Tryptophan, serotonin and hydroxyindole acetic acid levels in rat brain following slow or fast frequency electrostimulation. IRCS Med Sci 1982;10:427–8.

46 Capel ID, Pinnock MH, Patterson MA. The influence of electrostimulation on hexobarbital induced loss of righting reflex in rats. Acupuncture and Electro-Therapeutics Res, Int J 1982;7:17–26.

47 Capel ID, Pinnock MH, Withey NJ, Williams DC, Patterson MA. The effect of electrostimulation on barbiturate-induced sleeping times in rats. Drug Dev Res 1982;2:73–9.

48 Capel ID, Williams DC, Patterson MA. The amelioration of restraint stress by electrostimulation. IRCS Med Sci 1979;7:634.

49 Cara M, Debras C, Dufour B, Limoge A. Long-term electromedical anaesthesia in forty cases of major urological surgery. In: Wageneder FM, Germann RH, eds. Electrotherapeutic Sleep and Electroanaesthesia. Vol. III. Third International Symposium in Varna. Graz: RM Verlag, 1974.

50 Carney MWP, Bacelle L, Robinson B. Psychosis after cannabis abuse. Br Med J 1984;288:1047.

51 Catalan J, Gath DH. Benzodiazepines in general practice: time for a decision. Br Med J 1985;290:1374–6.

52 Catlin DH, Hui KK, Loh HH, Li CH. Pharmacologic activity of β-endorphin in man. Communications in Psychopharmacology 1977;1:493–500.

53 Charney DS, Sternberg DE, Kleber HD, Heninger GR, Redmond DE. The clinical use of clonidine in abrupt withdrawal from methadone. Arch Gen Psychiatry 1981;38:1273–7.

54 Cheng RSS, Pomeranz B, Yu G. Electroacupuncture treatment of morphine-dependent mice reduces signs of withdrawal without showing cross-tolerance. Eur J Pharmacol 1980;68:477.

55 Ch'ien J. Conversation with James Ch'ien. Br J Addiction 1981;76:3–8.

56 Chudecki P. Teenagers face new smoking crackdown. The Times 1984 July 23:1(cols 7–8).

57 Clement-Jones V, McLoughlin L, Lowry PJ, Besser GM, Rees LH, Wen HL. Acupuncture in heroin addicts: Changes in met-enkephalin and beta-endorphin in blood and cerebrospinal fluid. Lancet 1979;ii:380-2.

58 Clement-Jones V, Tomlin S, Rees LH, McLoughlin L, Besser GM, Wen HL. Increased β-endorphin but not met-enkephalin levels in human cerebrospinal fluid after acupuncture for recurrent pain. Lancet 1980;ii:946-9.

59 Clow A, Glover V, Armando I, Sandler M. New endogenous benzodiazepine receptor ligand in human urine: identity with endogenous monoamine oxidase inhibitor? Life Sciences 1983;33:735-41.

60 Cocteau Jean. Opium: the Diary of an Addict. New York: Grove Press, 1958.

61 Cohen S. Abuse of inhalants. In: Pradhan SN, Dutta SN, eds. Drug abuse. Clinical and basic aspects. Saint Louis: The CV Mosby Company, 1977:290-302.

62 Cohen S. The Substance Abuse Problems. New York: The Haworth Press, 1981:80.

63 Coleman Vernon. The Medicine Men: Drug makers, Doctors and Patients. New York: Transatlantic Arts Inc, 1977.

64 Collier HOJ. The experimental analysis of drug dependence. ICI (Imperial Chemical Industries) 1972 Sep.

65 Committee on the Review of Medicines. On benzodiazepines. Drug and Therapeutics Bulletin 1980;18:97.

66 Cook AW, Weinstein SP. Chronic dorsal column stimulation in M.S. NY State J Med 1973 Dec 15:2868-72.

67 Cooper IS, Riklan M, Snider RS, eds. The Cerebellum, Epilepsy and Behavior. New York: Plenum Press, 1974.

68 Ibid:119-71.

69 Ibid:217-27.

70 Ibid:229-44.

71 Cottrell D, Childs-Clarke A, Ghodse AH. British opiate addicts; an 11-year follow-up. Br J Psychiatry 1985;146:448-50.

72 Cousins Norman. Anatomy of an Illness. New York: WW Norton and Company, 1979.

73 Cowe L, Lloyd DJ, Dawling S. Neonatal convulsions caused by withdrawal from maternal clomipramine. Br Med J 1982;284:1837-8.

74 Cowen PJ, Nutt DJ. Abstinence symptoms after withdrawal of tranquillising drugs: is there a common neurochemical mechanism. Lancet 1982;ii:360-2.

75 Crime Incorporated Programme. Independent Television Channel 3, 1984 Sep 5.

76 Cronk SL, Barkley DEH, Farrell MF. Respiratory arrest after solvent abuse. Br Med J 1985;290:897-8.

77 Cubeddu LX, Hoffmann IS. Frequency-dependent release of acetylcholine and dopamine from rabbit striatum: its modulation by dopamine receptors. J Neurochemistry 1983;41:94-101.

78 Curtis DR, Eccles JC. Synaptic action during and after repetitive stimulation. J Physiol 1960;150:374-98.

79 Curzon G, Fernando JCR, Marsden CA. 5-hydroxytryptamine: the effects of impaired synthesis on its metabolism and release in rat. Br J Pharmacol 1978;63:627-34.

80 Cushman P. Detoxification of methadone maintained patients. In: Schecter A, Alksne H, Kaufman E, eds. Drug abuse: modern trends, issues and perspectives. New York: Marcel Decker, Inc, 1978;337-45.

81 Cushman P. Narcotic antagonists in the treatment of opiate dependency. Advances in Alcohol and Substance Abuse 1982;2:87-99.

82 Dackis CA, Gurpegui M, Pottash ALC, Gold MS. Methadone induced hypoadrenalism. Lancet 1982;ii:1167.

83 Davies W, Gonzales JP, Sewell RDe, Spencer PSJ. The effects of some antidepressants on the induction of morphine dependence and the morphine withdrawal syndrome. Alcohol and Alcoholism 1983;18:343-51.

84 Deitch R. Commentary from Westminster. Drug addiction. Lancet 1984; i:1029-30.

85 De Leon G. The role of rehabilitation. In: Nahas GG, Frick HC, eds. Drug abuse in the modern world. A perspective for the eighties. New York: Pergamon Press, 1981:298-307.

86 De Leon G, Wexler HK, Jainchill N. The therapeutic community: success and improvement rates 5 years after treatment. The Internat J Addictions 1982;17(4):703-47.

87 Demarest M. Cocaine: middle class high. Time 1981 July 6:56-63.

88 Dixey R, Rein G. H-noradrenaline release potentiated in a clonal nerve cell line by low-intensity pulsed magnetic fields. Nature 1982;296:253-6.

89 Dole VP, Nyswander ME. Methadone maintenance treatment: A ten-year perspective. JAMA 1976;235:2117-9.

90 Drink and drugs: double standards. The Economist 1982 Dec 4:33-4.

91 Drinking up time (Editorial). Observer 1984 Oct 7:8(cols 1-2).

92 Drug abuse. Shooting up. Economist 1984 Aug 18:25.

93 Drugs in Pakistan. In a fix. Economist 1984 June 16:41.

94 Dymond AM, Coger RW, Serafetinides EA. Intracerebral current levels in man during electro-sleep therapy. Biolog Psychiatry 1975;10:101-4.

95 Eady B. Kids, drugs and alcohol. USA Today 1983 April 25:1A(cols 6-7).

96 Eames L. The saving of Bernard. Sunday Times 1984 Feb 19:46(cols 1-5).

97 Edwards G, Busch C. The partnership between research and policy. In: Edwards G, Busch C, eds. Drug problems in Britain. London: Academic Press, 1981:314-5.

98 Edwards J Guy. Antidepressants - yes or no? Br Med J 1978;1:110.

99 Einstein S. Coping and drug misuse intervention (Editorial). International J Addictions 1984;19:iii-vii.

100 Ellinwood EH, Petrie WM. Dependence on amphetamine, cocaine and other stimulants. In: Pradhan SN, Dutta SN, eds. Drug abuse. Clinical and basic aspects. Saint Louis: The CV Mosby Company, 1977:248-62.

101 Essig C. Barbiturate dependence. In: Harris RT, McIsaac WM, Schuster CR, eds. Advances in mental science II. Austin and London: University of Texas Press, 1970;129-40.

102 Fang HSY. Must drug abuse be endemic in a modern society? - Problems and areas of cooperation in the Pan Pacific region. In: Stumpf KL, Chien JMN, MacQuarrie L, Oram W, Lam I, Lam E, eds. Towards a coordinated approach: current issues & future

directions. Hong Kong: Organising Committee for the 2nd Pan Pacific Conference on Drugs & Alcohol, 1985:3-6.

103 Fox EJ, Melzack R. Transcutaneous electrical stimulation and acupuncture: comparison of treatment for low-back pain. Pain 1976;2:141-8.

104 Frankl Victor. The Doctor and the Soul: from Psychotherapy to Logotherapy. New York: Vintage Books, 1977.

105 Frankl Victor. Man's Search for Meaning: an introduction to logotherapy. New York: Pocket Books, 1963.

106 Frederickson RCA. Morphine withdrawal response and central cholinergic activity. Nature 1975;257:131-2.

107 Freemantle Brian. The Fix. London: Michael Joseph Ltd, 1985.

108 Friedenberg ZB, Brighton CT. Electrical fracture healing. Ann NY Acad Sci 1974;238:564-74.

109 Galanter M, Diamond LC. Relief of psychiatric symptoms in evangelical religious sects. Br J Hosp Med 1981;Nov:495-8.

110 Gallacher S. George Patterson on drug addiction and rehabilitation. Radix 1981;13:3-8.

111 Giesler GJ, Liebeskind JC. Inhibition of visceral pain by electrical stimulation of the periaqueductal grey matter. Pain 1976;2:43-8.

112 Gintzler AR, Jaffe BM, Baron SA. Direct quantitation of the release of substance P from the myenteric plexus. In: Skrabanek P, Powell D, eds. Proceedings of the International Symposium on Substance P. Dublin: Boole Press, 1983:245-6.

113 Glover V, Clow A, Elsworth J, Sandler M. Tribulin in anxiety and panic. Clin Neuropharmacology 1984;7:178-9.

114 Godec C, Cass AS, Ayala GF. Electrical stimulation for incontinence. Technique, selection and results. Urology 1976;7:388-97.

115 Gold MS, Pottash AC. Endorphins, locus coeruleus, clonidine and lofexidine; a mechanism for opiate withdrawal and new nonopiate treatments. Advances in Alcohol and Substance Abuse 1981;1:33-52.

116 Gold MS, Pottash AC, Sweeney DR, Kleber HD, Redmond DE. Rapid opiate detoxification: clinical evidence of antidepressant and antipanic effects of opiates. Am J Psychiatry 1979;136:982-3.

117 Gold MS, Rea WS. The role of endorphins in opiate addiction, opiate withdrawal, and recovery. Psychiatric Clinics of N America 1983;6:1-32.

118 Golding J. Smoking - a way to control arousal? The Journal (The Addiction Research Foundation of Ontario) 1981 March 10:4.

119 Goldstein A. Heroin addiction. Sequential treatments employing pharmacologic supports. Arch Gen Psychiatry 1976;33:353-8.

120 Goldstein A, Hilgard ER. Failure of the opiate antagonist naloxone to modify hypnotic analgesia. Proc Nat Acad Sci 1975;72:2041-5.

121 Gomez E, Mikhail AR. Treatment of methadone withdrawal with cerebral electrotherapy (electrosleep). Br J Psychiatry 1979;134:111-13.

122 Goodman SJ, Holcombe V. Paper given at First World Congress on Pain. Florence, Italy, 1975.

123 Graeff FG, Quintero S, Gray JA. Median raphe stimulation, hippocampal theta rhythm and threat-induced behavioral inhibition. Physiol Behav 1980;25:253-61.

124 Griffin N, Draper RJ, Webb MGT. Addiction to tranylcypromine. Br Med J 1981;283:346.

125 Guillemin R, Vargo T, Rossier J, et al. Beta-endorphin and adrenocorticotropin are secreted concomitantly by the pituitary gland. Science 1977;197:1367-9.

126 Hall R. Police fight the Mandies. Observer 1984 Oct 7:6(col 9).

127 Hartnoll RL, Mitcheson MC, Battersby A, et al. Evaluation of heroin maintenance in controlled trial. Arch Gen Psychiatry 1980;37:877-84.

128 Hatterer L. Hard research strategies and soft clinical studies: comparative cross-cultural etiologies of the addictive process. In: Stumpf KL, Chien JMN, MacQuarrie L, Oram W, Lam I, Lam E, eds. Towards a coordinated approach: current issues & future directions. Hong Kong: Organizing Committee for the 2nd Pan Pacific Conference on Drugs & Alcohol, 1985:249-56.

129 Herz A, Duka T, Gramsch C, et al. Pharmacologic manipulation of brain and pituitary endorphin content and release. In: Costa E, Trabucchi M, eds. Neural Peptides and Neuronal Communication. New York: Raven Press, 1980:323-33.

130 Himmelsbach CK. Clinical studies of drug addiction. Physical dependence, withdrawal and recovery. Arch Intern Med 1942;69:766–72.

131 Ho WKK, Wen HL, Ling N. Beta-endorphin-like immunoactivity in the plasma of heroin addicts and normal subjects. Neuropharmacology 1980;19:117–20.

132 Hoffmann. Quoted by Lawrie P. In: Drugs: Medical, Psychological and Social Facts. London: Penguin 1974.

133 Hosobuchi Y, Rossier J, Bloom FE, Guillemin R. Stimulation of human periaqueductal grey for pain relief increases immunoreactive β-endorphin in ventricular fluid. Science 1979;203:279–81.

134 House of Commons Official Report 1984 April:656.

135 Ibid May: 1463.

136 Ibid July:1441–2.

137 Ibid:1450.

138 Ibid:1455–60.

139 Ibid:1470.

140 Ibid:1479–81.

141 Ibid:1499–500.

142 Ibid:1506.

143 Howlett TA, Tomlin S, Ngahfoong L, et al. Release of β-endorphin and met-enkephalin during exercise in normal women: response to training. Br Med J 1984;288:1950–2.

144 Hughes J. Enkephalin and drug dependence. Br J Addiction 1976;71:199–209.

145 Hughes J. Isolation of an endogenous compound from the brain with pharmacological properties similar to morphine. Brain Res 1975;88:295–306.

146 Hughes J, Smith TW, Morgan B, Fothergill L. Purification and properties of enkephalin – the possible endogenous ligand for the morphine receptor. Life Sci 1975;16:1753–8.

147 Huprich ST. Doctoral Dissertation, University of California at Los Angeles, 1975. Quoted by Liebeskind et al, 1976.

148 Huw J, Morgan C. Addiction to tranylcypromine. Br Med J 1981;283:618.

149 Hynes MD, Lockner MA, Bemis KG, Hymson DL. Chronic ethanol alters the receptor binding characteristics of the delta opioid receptor ligand, D-Ala^2-D-Leu^5 enkephalin in mouse-brain. Life Sciences 1983;33:2331-7.

150 Illis LS. Experimental model of regeneration in the central nervous system. Brain 1973;96:47-60.

151 Illis LS, Sedgwick EM, Oygar AE, Sabbahi Awadalla MA. Dorsal-column stimulation in the rehabilitation of patients with multiple sclerosis. Lancet 1976; i:1383-6.

152 Inaba D. Needle therapy. The New York Times 1982 March 14:49(cols 2-4).

153 Iversen LL. Neurotransmitters and CNS disease. Lancet 1982; ii:914-18.

154 Jamrozik K, Fowler G, Vessey M, Wald N. Placebo controlled trial of nicotine chewing gum in general practice. Br Med J 1984;289:794-7.

155 Janal MN, Colt EWD, Clark WC, Glusman M. Pain sensitivity, mood, and plasma endocrine levels in man following long-distance running; effects of naloxone. Pain 1984;19:13-25.

156 John ER, Kleinman D. 'Stimulus generalization' between differentiated visual, auditory and central stimuli. J Neurophysiol 1975;38:1015-34.

157 Jones CJ, Wilson SM. The effect of autonomic agonists and nerve stimulation on protein secretion from the rat submandibular gland. J Physiol 1985;358:65-73.

158 Jones I, Simpson D, Brown AC, Bainton D, McDonald H. Prescribing psychotropic drugs in general practice: three year study. Br Med J 1984;289:1045-8.

159 Jung Carl. Ed. Man and His Symbols. New York: Doubleday and Company Inc, 1964.

160 Jung Carl. Memories, Dreams, Reflections. Recorded and ed. by Aniela Jaffe. New York: Pantheon Books, 1963.

161 Jung Carl. Modern Man in Search of a Soul. New York: Harcourt, Brace and Company, 1933.

162 Kaada B. Neurophysiological mechanisms of pain suppression and cutaneous vasodilation induced by transcutaneous nerve stimulation (TNS) and acupuncture – a review. Legevitenskap og livsvisdom. Festschrift to Tollak B Sirnes on his 60th anniversary. 1982:64–94.

163 Kaada B. Promoted healing of chronic ulceration by transcutaneous nerve stimulation (TNS). VASA 1983;12:262–9.

164 Kaada B. Vasodilation induced by transcutaneous nerve stimulation in peripheral ischaemia (Raynaud's phenomenon and diabetic polyneuropathy). Europ Heart J 1982;3:303–14.

165 Kaada B, Eielsen O. In search of mediators of skin vasodilation induced by transcutaneous nerve stimulation: II Serotonin implicated. Gen Pharmacol 1983;14:635–41.

166 Kales A, Malmstrom EJ, Rickles WH, et al. Sleep patterns of a pentobarbital addict: before and after withdrawal. Psychophysiology 1968;5:208.

167 Kales A, Scharf MB, Kales JD. Rebound insomnia: a new clinical syndrome. Science 1978;201:1039–41.

168 Kawakita K, Funakoshi M. Suppression of the jaw-opening reflex by conditioning A-delta fiber stimulation and electroacupuncture in the rat. Experimental Neurology 1982;78:461–5.

169 Keerdoja A, Aubenow GC, Abramson P, McColl C. How to win a losing battle. Newsweek 1982 Dec 13:18–22.

170 Kelleher RT. Psychomotor stimulants. In: Pradhan SN, Dutta SN, eds. Drug abuse. Clinical and basic aspects. Saint Louis: The CV Mosby Company, 1977:116–47.

171 Kelsey Morton. (Quoting Jung). Encounter with God. Minneapolis: Bethany Fellowship Inc, 1972.

172 Key DC. Human sleep during chronic morphine detoxification. Psychopharmacologia 1975;44:117–24.

173 Koestler Arthur, Smythies JR. Beyond Reductionism: Alpbach Symposium 1968. New York: Macmillan, 1970.

174 Kolb L, Himmelsbach CK. A critical review of the withdrawal treatments with method of evaluating abstinence syndromes. Am J Psychiatry 1938;94:759–99.

175 Kort J, Ito H, Bassett CAL. Effects of pulsing electromagnetic fields (PEMF's) on peripheral nerve regeneration. 26th Annual Orthopaedic Research Symposium, Atlanta, Georgia, 1980. Quoted

in: Binder A, Parr G, Hazleman B, Fitton-Jackson S. Pulsed electromagnetic field therapy of persistent rotator cuff tendinitis. A double-blind controlled assessment. Lancet 1984;i:695–8.

176 Kosterlitz HW, Hughes J. Some thoughts on the significance of enkephalin, the endogenous ligand. Life Sci 1975;17:91–6.

177 Kosterlitz HW, Paterson SJ. Characterisation of opioid receptors in nervous tissue. Proc Roy Soc B 1980;210:113–22.

178 Kuhar MJ, Pert CB, Snyder SH. Regional distribution of opiate receptor binding in monkey and human brain. Nature 1973;245:447–50.

179 Lader M. Address to the Centennial Symposium of the Society for the Study of Addiction at the Royal Society. 1984 Oct 25–6.

180 Law W, Petti TA, Kazdin AE. Withdrawal symptoms after graduated cessation of imipramine in children. Am J Psychiatry 1981;138:647–50.

181 Lawrie Peter. Drugs: Medical, Psychological and Social Facts. London: Penguin, 1974.

182 Let them smoke pot. Economist 1984 Jan 28:51.

183 Levine JD, Gordon NC, Fields HL. The mechanism of placebo analgesia. Lancet 1978;ii:654–7.

184 Lewis RV, Stern AS, Kimura S, et al. Opioid peptides and precursors in the adrenal medulla. In: Costa E, Trabucchi M, eds. Neural Peptides and Neuronal Communication. New York: Raven Press, 1980:167–79.

185 Lewis SA, Oswald I, Evans JI, Akindale MO, Tompsett SL. Heroin and human sleep. Electroenceph Clin Neurophysiolog 1970;28:374–81.

186 Liberation Daily News 1972 Jan 22.

187 Liebeskind JC, Giesler GJ, Urca G. Evidence pertaining to an endogenous mechanism of pain inhibition in the central nervous system. In: Zotterman Y, ed. Sensory functions of the skin in primates, with special reference to man. Oxford: Pergamon Press, 1976.

188 Liebeskind JC, Guilbaud G, Besson JM, Oliveras JL. Analgesia from electrical stimulation of the periaqueductal grey matter in the cat: behavioral observations and inhibitory effects on spinal cord interneurons. Brain Res 1973;50:441–6.

189 Liebman JM, Mayer DJ, Liebeskind JC. Mesencephalic central grey lesions and fear-motivated behavior in rats. Brain Res 1970;23:353-70.

190 Limoge A, Debras C, Coeytaux R, Cara M. Electrical technique for electropharmaceutical anaesthesia concerning 300 operations. In: Wageneder FM, Germann RH, eds. Electrotherapeutic Sleep and Electroanaesthesia. Graz: RM Verlag, 1975.

191 Lipton DS, Maranda MJ. Detoxification from heroin dependency: an overview of method and effectiveness. Advances in Alcohol and Substance Abuse 1982;2:31-55.

192 Lister RG, File SE. The nature of lorazepam-induced amnesia. Psychopharmacology 1984;83:183-7.

193 Lloyd G. I am an alcoholic. Br Med J 1982;285:785-6.

194 Long DM, Hagfors N. Electrical stimulation in the nervous system: the current status of electrical stimulation of the nervous system for relief of pain. Brain 1975;1:109-23.

195 Lovick TA, Wolstencroft JH. Actions of GABA, glycine, methionine-enkephalin and β-endorphin compared with electrical stimulation of nucleus raphe magnus on responses evoked by tooth pulp stimulation in the medial reticular formation in the cat. Pain 1983;15:131-44.

196 Lucchi L, Rius RA, Uzumaki H, Govoni S, Trabucchi M. Chronic ethanol changes opiate receptor function in rat striatum. Brain Research 1984;293:368-71.

197 Madden JS. Alcohol and drug dependence: areas of change or uncertainty. Alcohol and Alcoholism 1983;18:305-12.

198 Mann Felix. Acupuncture: Cure of Many Diseases. London: William Heinemann Medical Books. 1972.

199 Mao W, Ghia JN, Scott DS, Duncan GH, Gregg JM. High versus low intensity acupuncture analgesia for treatment of chronic pain: effects on platelet serotonin. Pain 1980;8:331-42.

200 Marlatt GA, Rohsenow DJ. The think-drink effect. Psychology Today 1981;Dec:60-9.

201 Martin WR. Dependence on narcotic analgesics. In: Pradhan SN, Dutta SN, eds. Drug abuse. Clinical and basic aspects. Saint Louis: The CV Mosby Company, 1977;201-10.

202 Masi D (interview). Drugs cost industry $25 billion each year. USA Today 1983 March 10:11A(cols 1-7).

203 Matatu G. 'Mandrax trail' drug smugglers foiled by gold. Observer 1984 Oct 14:13(cols 1-2).

204 May Rollo. Love and Will. New York: WW Norton and Company Inc, 1969.

205 Mayer DJ. Pain inhibition by electrical brain stimulation: comparison to morphine. Neurosci Res Prog Bull 1975;13:94-100.

206 Mayer DJ, Liebeskind JC. Pain reduction by focal electric stimulation of the brain - an anatomical and behavioral analysis. Brain Res 1974;68:73-93.

207 Mayer DJ, Wolffe TL, Akil H, Carder B, Liebeskind JC. Analgesia from electrical stimulation in the brainstem of the rat. Science 1971;174:1351-4.

208 McGeer PL, Eccles Sir John C, McGeer EG. Molecular Neurobiology of the Mammalian Brain. New York and London: Plenum Press, 1978:199-231.

209 McIlvanney H. Greaves gets by on his own spirit. Observer 1984 Oct 7:38(cols 1-8).

210 Melzack R. The Puzzle of Pain. New York: Basic Books Inc, 1973.

211 Melzack R, Stillwell DM, Fox EJ. Trigger points and acupuncture points for pain: correlations and implications. Pain 1977;3:3-23.

212 Meyer F. Evidence before hearing of California State Senate Health Committee. The Journal (The Addiction Research Foundation of Ontario) 1977 March 1:6(3),5.

213 Minegishi A, Fukumori R, Satch T, Kitagawa H, Yanaura S. Interaction of lithium and disulfiram in hexobarbital hypnosis: possible role of the 5-HT system. J Pharmacol Experimental Therapeutics 1981;218:481-7.

214 Mitcheson M, Hartnoll R. Conflicts in deciding treatment within drug dependency clinics. In: West DJ, ed. Problems of drug abuse in Britain. Cambridge: Institute of Criminology, 1978:74-8.

215 Moore RA. Dependence on alcohol. In: Pradhan SN, Dutta SN, eds. Drug abuse. Clinical and basic aspects. Saint Louis: The CV Mosby Company, 1977;211-29.

216 Murray RM. Alcoholism and employment. J of Alcoholism 1975;10:23-6.

217 Nathan PW, Wall PD. Treatment of post-herpetic neuralgia by prolonged electric stimulation. Br Med J 1974;3:645–7.

218 National Strategy for Prevention of Drug Abuse and Drug Trafficking. Drug Abuse Policy Office: The White House, 1984:26.

219 Ng LKY, Douthitt TO, Thoa NB, Albert CA. Modification of morphine-withdrawal syndrome in rats following transauricular electrostimulation: an experimental paradigm for auricular electroacupuncture. Biolog Psychiatry 1975;10:575–80.

220 Ng LKY, Szara S, Bunney WE. On understanding and treating narcotic dependence: a neuropsychopharmacological perspective. Br J Addiction 1975;70:311–24.

221 Nias DKB. Therapeutic effects of low-level direct electrical currents. Psychol Bull 1976;83:766–73.

222 Nicholi AM. The nontherapeutic use of psychoactive drugs. A modern epidemic. N Engl J Med 1983;308:925–33.

223 NIDA Research Monograph Series 25: Behavioral Analysis and Treatment of Substance Abuse. Washington DC: Government Printing Office, 1979. Quoted from Peele S. How Much Is Too Much, 1981:86.

224 Nordenström BEW. Biologically Closed Electric Circuits. Stockholm, Sweden: Nordic Medical Publications, 1983:281–316.

225 Oliveras JL, Redjemi F, Guilbaud G, Besson JM. Analgesia induced by electrical stimulation of the inferior centralis nucleus of the raphe in the cat. Pain 1975;1:139–45.

226 1983 Jan by Omni Publications International Ltd and reprinted with the permission of the copyright owner.

227 One million pounds extra for drug abuse is 'derisory'. The Guardian 1984 July 14:3(cols 1–2).

228 O'Reilly. New insights into alcoholism. Time 1983 April 25:88–9.

229 Orwell G. Notes on Nationalism. Polemic 1945 Oct.

230 Oswald I, Evans JI, Lewis SA. Addictive drugs cause suppression of paradoxical sleep with withdrawal rebound. In: Steinberg Hannah, ed. Scientific Basis of Drug Dependence. London: Churchill, 1969.

231 Parish P. Medicines. A guide for everybody. New York: Penguin Books, 1979:44–5.

232 Ibid: 47-50.

233 Pasternak GW, Goodman R, Snyder SH. An endogenous morphine-like factor in mammalian brain. Life Sci 1975;16:1765-9.

234 Paton A. The politics of alcohol. Br Med J 1985;290:1-2.

235 Patterson George N. Christianity and Marxism. Exeter, England: Paternoster Press, 1982.

236 Patterson MA. Acupuncture and neuroelectric therapy in the treatment of drug and alcohol addictions. Aust J Alc Drug Dependence 1975;2:90-5.

237 Patterson MA. Addictions Can Be Cured. Berkhamsted, England: Lion Publishing, 1975:92.

238 Patterson MA. Effects of NeuroElectric Therapy (NET) in drug addiction: an interim report. UN Bull Narc 1976;28:55-62.

239 Patterson MA. Electro-acupuncture in alcohol and drug addictions. Clin Med 1974;81:9-13.

240 Patterson MA. NeuroElectric Therapy: are endorphins involved? Mim's Magazine 1981 Sep:22-5.

241 Patterson MA. The significance of current frequency in NeuroElectric Therapy (NET) for drug and alcohol addictions. In: Wageneder FM, Germann RH, eds. Electrotherapeutic Sleep and Electroanaesthesia. Graz: RM Verlag, 1978:285-96.

242 Patterson MA, Firth J, Gardiner R. Treatment of drug, alcohol and nicotine addiction by NeuroElectric Therapy: analysis of results over 7 years. J Bioelectricity 1984;3:193-221.

243 Peele S. How Much Is Too Much. Healthy habits or destructive addictions. Englewood Cliffs NJ: Prentice-Hall Inc, 1981.

244 Peele Stanton. Love and Addiction. New York: Taplinger Publishing Company Inc, 1975.

245 Pert CB, Snyder SH. Opiate receptor: demonstration in nervous tissue. Science 1973;179:1011-4.

246 Peturrson H, Lader MH. Withdrawal reaction from clobazepam. Br Med J 1981;282:1931-2.

247 Peturrson H, Bhattacharya SK, Glover V, Sandler M, Lader MH. Urinary monoamine oxidase inhibitor and benzodiazepine withdrawal. Br J Psychiatry 1982;140:7-10.

248 Picardie J, Rosselli M. 'The thin blue line has snapped'. Sunday Times 1984 June 3:9(cols 4-6).

249 Pisani VD. Clinical implications of neuropsychological impairment in alcoholics. In: Stumpf KL, Chien JMN, MacQuarrie L, Oram W, Lam I, Lam E, eds. Towards a coordinated approach: current issues & future directions. Hong Kong: Organizing Committee for the 2nd Pan Pacific Conference on Drugs & Alcohol, 1985:225-31.

250 Pomeranz B, Mullen M, Markus H. Effect of applied electrical fields on sprouting of intact saphenous nerve in adult rat. Brain Research 1984;303:331-6.

251 Pounds 3.7 million granted for drug services. ISDD Druglink 1984;19(Spring):30.

252 Power KG, Jerrom DWA, Simpson RJ, Mitchell M. Controlled study of withdrawal symptoms and rebound anxiety after six week course of diazepam for generalised anxiety. Br Med J 1985;290:1246-8.

253 Prevention. Report of the Advisory Council on the Misuse of Drugs. H M Stationery Office, 1984:85.

254 Pullan PT, Watson FE, Seow SSW, Rappeport W. Methadone-induced hypoadrenalism. Lancet 1983;i:714.

255 Quirion R, DiMaggio DA, French ED, et al. Evidence for an endogenous peptide ligand for the phencyclidine receptor. Peptides 1984;5:967-73.

256 Raji ARM, Bowen REM. Effects of high peak pulsed electromagnetic field on degeneration and regeneration of the common peroneal nerve in rats. Lancet 1982;ii:444-5.

257 Ramos A, Schwartz EL, Roy JE. Stable and plastic unit discharge patterns during behavioral generalization. Science 1976;192:393-6.

258 Report of the Medical Working Group on Drug Dependence. Guidelines of good clinical practice in the treatment of drug misuse. London: DHSS, 1984:19-21.

259 Ibid:10.

260 Research Committee of the British Thoracic Society. Comparison of four methods of smoking withdrawal in patients with smoking related diseases. Br Med J 1983;286:595-7.

261 Research Group of Acupuncture Anaesthesia, Peking Medical College. The role of some neurotransmitters of brain in finger-acupuncture analgesia. Scientia Sinica 1974;17:112-30.

262 Response to the treatment and rehabilitation report. ISSD Druglink 1984;19(Spring):16–7.

263 Ibid:18.

264 Ibid:20.

265 Rhodes DL. Doctoral Dissertation, University of California at Los Angeles, 1975. Quoted by Liebeskind et al, 1976.

266 Richardson DE, Akil H. Paper given at 7th Annual Meeting of the Neuroelectric Society, 1974. Quoted by Liebeskind et al, 1976.

267 Roberts JL. Campus binge. Wall Street Journal 1983 Feb 8:1(col 1),21(cols 1–3).

268 Rogers HJ, Specter RG, Trounce JR. A Textbook of Clinical Pharmacology. London: Hodder and Stoughton, 1981:193–279.

269 Rosenthal SH. Electrosleep: a double-blind study. Biolog Psychiatry 1972;4:179–85.

270 Rosenthal SH, Calvert LF. Electrosleep: personal subjective experiences. Biolog Psychiatry 1972;4:187–90.

271 Rosenthal SH, Wulfsohn NL. Electrosleep – a clinical trial. Am J Psychiatry 1970;127:175–6.

272 Rosenthal SH, Wulfsohn NL. Electrosleep – a preliminary communication. J Nerv Ment Dis 1970;151:146–51.

273 Rossier J, French E, Guillemin R, Bloom FE. On the mechanisms of the simultaneous release of immunoreactive β-endorphin, ACTH, and prolactin by stress. In: Costa E, Trabucchi M, eds. Neural Peptides and Neuronal Communication. New York: Raven Press, 1980:363–75.

274 Roubicek J, Zaks A, Freedman AM. EEG changes produced by heroin and methadone. Electroencephalogr Clin Neurophysiol 1969;27:667–8.

275 Rowley BA, McKenna JM, Chase GR, Wolcott LE. The influence of electrical current on an infecting microorganism in wounds. Ann NY Acad Sci 1974;238:543–51.

276 Russell M. Address to the Centennial Symposium of the Society for the Study of Addiction at The Royal Society. 1984 Oct 25–6.

277 Ryan JJ. Effects of transcerebral electrotherapy (electrosleep) on state anxiety according to suggestibility levels. Biolog Psychiatry 1976;11:233–8.

278 Salar G, Job I, Mingrino S, Bosio A, Trabucchi M. Effects of transcutaneous electrotherapy on CSF β-endorphin content in patients without pain problems. Pain 1981;10:169–72.

279 Salmons S, Sreter FA. Significance of impulse activity in the transformation of skeletal muscle type. Nature 1976; 263:30–4.

280 Sarai K, Kayano M. The level and diurnal rhythm of serum serotonin in manic-depressive patients. Folia Psychiatry Neurol Japan 1968;22:271–8.

281 Science Report. The Times 1974 March 28.

282 Sclare AB. Alcoholism in doctors. Br J on Alcohol and Alcoholism 1979;14:181–96.

283 Selye Hans. Stress Without Distress. Philadelphia, PA: JB Lippincott and Company, 1974.

284 Shapiro J. Nicotine chewing gum in general practice. Br Med J 1984;289:1308.

285 Simpson DD. Treatment for drug abuse. Follow-up outcomes and length of time spent. Arch Gen Psychiatry 1981;38:875–80.

286 Simpson DD, Savage LJ. Drug abuse treatment readmissions and outcomes. Three-year follow-up of DARP patients. Arch Gen Psychiatry 1980;37:896–901.

287 Sjölund BH, Eriksson MBE. The influence of naloxone on analgesia produced by peripheral conditioning stimulation. Brain Res 1979;173:295–301.

288 Sjölund B, Terenius L, Eriksson M. Increased cerebrospinal fluid levels of endorphins after electro-acupuncture. Acta Physiol Scand 1977;100:382–4.

289 Smith Adam. Powers of Mind. New York: Randon House Inc, 1975.

290 Smith CM. Pathophysiology of the alcohol withdrawal syndrome. Medical Hypotheses 1981;7:231–49.

291 Smyth DK. Morphine-like peptides in the brain. Sandoz Foundation Lecture, Institute of Neurology, London, 1976.

292 Solzhenitsyn A. From Under the Rubble. South Bend IA: Regnery-Gateway Inc, 1981.

293 Spotts JV, Shontz FC. Drug-induced ego states. I. Cocaine: phenomenology and implications. International J Addictions 1984;19:119–151.

294 Stadelmayr-Maiyores HG. Technique of electrosleep therapy I. In: Wageneder FM, Germann RH, eds. Electrotherapeutic Sleep and Electroanaesthesia. Vol III. Third International Symposium in Varna. Graz: RM Verlag, 1974.

295 Sternbach RA, Janewsky DS, Huey LY, Segal DS. Effects of altering brain serotonin in activity on human chronic pain. In: Bonica JJ, Albe-Fessard D, eds. Advances in Pain Research and Therapy. Vol I. New York: Raven Press, 1976:601-6.

296 Stimmel B. Treatment for substance abuse: myths versus realities (Editorial). Advances in Alcohol and Substance Abuse 1982;2:1-6.

297 Stimson GV, Oppenheimer E. Heroin Addiction: Treatment and Control in Britain. London, New York: Tavistock Publications, 1982:212.

298 Ibid:216.

299 Ibid:231.

300 Ibid:236.

301 Stubbs DF. Frequency and the brain. Life Sci 1976;18:1-14.

302 Su CY, Lin CS, Peng C, et al. Suppression of morphine abstinence in heroin addicts by β-endorphin. In: Costa E, Trabucchi M, eds. Neural Peptides and Neuronal Communication. New York: Raven Press, 1980:503-9.

303 Supathan HR. Treatment of drug addicts by the traditional Malay medicine. In: Stumpf KL, Chien JMN, MacQuarrie L, Oram W, Lam I, Lam E, eds. Towards a coordinated approach: current issues & future directions. Hong Kong: Organizing Committee for the 2nd Pan Pacific Conference on Drugs & Alcohol, 1985:273-6.

304 Surveys and Statistics on Drugtaking in Britain. ISDD Library and Information Service 1983(March):6-7.

305 Sutherland EW. Dependence on barbiturates and other CNS depressants. In: Pradhan SN, Dutta SN, eds. Drug abuse. Clinical and basic aspects. Saint Louis: The CV Mosby Company, 1977;235-47.

306 Sweet WH, Wespic JG. Treatment of chronic pain by stimulation of fibres of primary afferent neurons. TransAmerica Neural Association 1968;93:103-7.

307 Szymanski HV. Prolonged depersonalisation after marijuana use. Am J Psychiatry 1981;138:231-3.

308 Temple Archbishop William. Readings from St. John's Gospel. London: Macmillan Publishers Ltd, 1961.

309 Tendler S. US drugs chief warns Britain of cocaine risk. The Times 1984 Dec 8:3(cols 1-2).

310 Tennant FS, Rawson RA, McCann M. Withdrawal from chronic Phencyclidine (PCP) dependence with desipramine. Am J Psychiatry 1981;138:845-7.

311 Terenius L, Wahlström A. Search for an endogenous ligand for the opiate receptor. Acta Physiol Scand 1975;94:74-81.

312 Tillich Paul. The Courage To Be. New Haven, Connecticut: Yale University Press, 1952.

313 Tillich Paul. The Meaning of Health. Richmond, California: North Atlantic Books, 1981;17-8,60.

314 The Times Diary. Rubbing shoulders. The Times 1984 Sep 5:12(col 1).

315 Timmins N. Heroin threatens fabric of society. The Times 1984 July 6:3(cols 7-8).

316 Tims FM. Evaluation of drug abuse treatment effectiveness: summary of the DARP followup research. Treatment Research Report for NIDA, 1982; DHSS publication no. (ADM)82-1194.

317 Tinklenberg JR. Abuse of marijuana. In: Pradhan SN, Dutta SN, eds. Drug abuse. Clinical and basic aspects. Saint Louis: The CV Mosby Company, 1977:268-73.

318 Tribulin - a natural panic molecule? New Scientist 1982 June 24:845.

319 Trickett SA. Coming Off Tranquillizers. Newcastle upon Tyne: SAT Publishing, 1985.

320 Trocchi Alex. Cain's Book. New York: Grove Press, 1960.

321 Troiani J. Report in The Journal 1981;10(11):4(cols 1-3).

322 Tyrer PJ. Benzodiazepines on trial. Br Med J 1984;288:1101-2.

323 Tyrer P, Owen R, Dawling S. Gradual withdrawal of diazepam after long-term therapy. Lancet 1983;i:1402-6.

324 Tyrer P, Rutherford D, Huggett T. Benzodiazepine withdrawal symptoms and propanolol. Lancet 1981;i:520-2.

325 US Government pamphlet. Why people smoke cigarettes. Los Angeles Times 1983 March 7:Part I,5(cols 5-6).

326 Vacca LL, Arakawa K, Naftchi NE, Guan X-M, Ai M. Immunocytochemical changes in peptides substance P and enkephalin in rat spinal cord after electroacupuncture. In: Skrabanek P, Powell D, eds. Proceedings of the International Symposium on Substance P. Dublin: Boole Press, 1983:208-9.

327 Vaillant GE. A 20-year follow-up of New York narcotic addicts. Arch Gen Psychiatry 1973;29:237-41.

328 Vaillant GE. The Natural History of Alcoholism. Cambridge, Mass and London: Harvard University Press, 1983:287,300,314.

329 van Praag HM. Depression. Lancet 1982;ii:1259-64.

330 van Ree JM. Neuropeptides and addictive behaviour. Alcohol and Alcoholism 1983;18:325-30.

331 Wagner MS. Getting the health out of people's daily lives. Lancet 1982;ii:1207-8.

332 Walker JB. Electrical stimulation enhanced recovery of function: how are peptides involved? Lancet 1983;ii:912.

333 Wall PD, Sweet WH. Temporary abolition of pain in man. Science 1967;155:108-9.

334 Walter W Grey. The Living Brain. London: Duckworth and Company, 1946.

335 Washton AM, Gold MS, Pottash AC. Intranasal cocaine addiction. Lancet 1983;ii:1374.

336 Washton AM, Gold MS, Pottash AC, Semlitz L. Adolescent cocaine abusers. Lancet 1984;ii:746.

337 Washton AM, Resnick RB. Clonidine in opiate withdrawal: review and appraisal of clinical findings. Pharmacotherapy 1981;1:140-6.

338 Wen HL, Chau K. Status asthmaticus treated by acupuncture and electrostimulation. Asian J Med 1973;9:191-2.

339 Wen HL, Cheung SY. Treatment of drug addiction by acupuncture and electrical stimulation. Asian J Med 1973;9:138-41.

340 Wen HL, Ho WKK, Ling N, Ma L, Choa GH. The influence of electroacupuncture on naloxone-induced morphine withdrawal. II. Elevation of immunoassayable beta-endorphin activity in the brain but not in the blood. Am J Chinese Med 1979;7:237-40.

341 Wen HL, Ng YH, Ho WKK, Fung KP, Wong HK, Wong HC. Acupuncture in narcotic withdrawal: a preliminary report on biochemical changes in the blood and urine of heroin addicts. Bull Narc 1978;30:31-9.

342 Wesson J. What do we do about Donny? Third Way 1984;7:20-2.

343 Wetli CV, Wright RF. Death caused by recreational cocaine use. JAMA 1979;241:2519-22.

344 Wille R. Ten-year follow-up of a representative sample of London heroin addicts: clinic attendance, abstinence and mortality. Br J Addiction 1981;76:259-66.

345 Wilson DH, Jagadeesh P. Experimental regeneration in peripheral nerves and the spinal cord in laboratory animals exposed to a pulsed electromagnetic field. Paraplegia 1976;14:12-20.

346 Wilson JQ. The fix. The New Republic 1982 Oct 25:24-9.

347 Wint Guy, ed. Asia Handbook. London: Blond and Briggs, 1965. London: Penguin Books, 1969.

348 Wint Guy. The Third Killer. London: Chatto and Windus, 1965.

349 Yang MMP, Kwok JSL. Evaluation on the treatment of morphine addiction by acupuncture, Chinese herbs and opioid peptides. Amer J of Chinese Medicine (in press).

350 Young J, Lerner MA, Dallas R, Widmann L, Stanger T. The white plague's toll. Newsweek 1984 Aug 13:12-3.

325 US Government pamphlet. Why people smoke cigarettes. Los Angeles Times 1983 March 7:Part I,5(cols 5-6).

326 Vacca LL, Arakawa K, Naftchi NE, Guan X-M, Ai M. Immunocytochemical changes in peptides substance P and enkephalin in rat spinal cord after electroacupuncture. In: Skrabanek P, Powell D, eds. Proceedings of the International Symposium on Substance P. Dublin: Boole Press, 1983:208-9.

327 Vaillant GE. A 20-year follow-up of New York narcotic addicts. Arch Gen Psychiatry 1973;29:237-41.

328 Vaillant GE. The Natural History of Alcoholism. Cambridge, Mass and London: Harvard University Press, 1983:287,300,314.

329 van Praag HM. Depression. Lancet 1982;ii:1259-64.

330 van Ree JM. Neuropeptides and addictive behaviour. Alcohol and Alcoholism 1983;18:325-30.

331 Wagner MS. Getting the health out of people's daily lives. Lancet 1982;ii:1207-8.

332 Walker JB. Electrical stimulation enhanced recovery of function: how are peptides involved? Lancet 1983;ii:912.

333 Wall PD, Sweet WH. Temporary abolition of pain in man. Science 1967;155:108-9.

334 Walter W Grey. The Living Brain. London: Duckworth and Company, 1946.

335 Washton AM, Gold MS, Pottash AC. Intranasal cocaine addiction. Lancet 1983;ii:1374.

336 Washton AM, Gold MS, Pottash AC, Semlitz L. Adolescent cocaine abusers. Lancet 1984;ii:746.

337 Washton AM, Resnick RB. Clonidine in opiate withdrawal: review and appraisal of clinical findings. Pharmacotherapy 1981;1:140-6.

338 Wen HL, Chau K. Status asthmaticus treated by acupuncture and electrostimulation. Asian J Med 1973;9:191-2.

339 Wen HL, Cheung SY. Treatment of drug addiction by acupuncture and electrical stimulation. Asian J Med 1973;9:138-41.

340 Wen HL, Ho WKK, Ling N, Ma L, Choa GH. The influence of electroacupuncture on naloxone-induced morphine withdrawal. II. Elevation of immunoassayable beta-endorphin activity in the brain but not in the blood. Am J Chinese Med 1979;7:237-40.

Appendix II
Notes

1 Dr David Ausubel of New York reported the effects of methadone maintenance treatment in 1983:

> The psychopharmacological rationale and clinical effectiveness of the methadone maintenance treatment program was subjected to critical theoretical and methodological analysis. It was concluded (1) that the MMTP constitutes and perpetuates an immature coping mechanism; i.e., 'subliminal euphoria' - pervasive pharmacological shielding of addicts from the inevitable discomforts attending adaptation to the real world; (2) that it does not satisfy so-called tissue craving for florid euphoria because most 'stabilised' clients actively seek and obtain same from heroin, methadone itself, and/or other potentially euphorogenic drugs; (3) that the source of this craving resides in the addict's personality rather than in his tissues; (4) that official evaluation studies of MMTP grossly exaggerate its clinical effectiveness; and (5) that the MMTP has inadvertently created incomparably more primary methadone addicts than it has cured heroin addicts.[22]

2 In his book, *The Puzzle of Pain*, discussing these and other findings, Dr Ronald Melzack describes the inhibitory effect that the central tegmental tract had on input:

> The inhibitory influence may help to explain an exciting recent discovery. Reynolds (1969, 1970) has observed that electrical stimulation in the region of the central grey and central tegmental tract produces a marked analgesia in rats, so that they fail to respond to pinch, burn, even major abdominal surgery ... More recently, Mayer, Akil and Liebeskind (1971) observed the same phenomenon, and found, moreover, that there is some somatotopic organization within the system, so that stimulation at a given site produces analgesia of only selected positions of the body, such as the lower half, or one quadrant. They found, furthermore, that the electrical sti-

> mulation of these areas appears 'pleasurable' to the animals – they actively seek it out by pressing a lever to stimulate themselves. These observations . . . have great theoretical significance since they suggest the presence of a system that exerts a tonic, widespread inhibitory influence on transmission through the somatosensory projection system.[210]

3 The 'gate-theory' of pain control was that it had been demonstrated physiologically that all pain information travels to the spinal cord via small unmyelinated C fibres and that stimulation of the larger myelinated A fibres was never painful. Further, activity in the large A fibres inhibited, at the first spinal synapse, immediate subsequent activity from the smallest fibres considered essential to pain conduction. Dr Wall and Dr Melzack suggested that this mechanism normally acted as a 'gate' to balance pain and non-pain input.

4 In 1970 an experiment conducted in the state of Kansas, USA, confirmed a revolutionary new medical theory that had been gaining currency for the previous few years – that many body functions thought to be involuntary could, in fact, be controlled. The experiment, conducted by Dr Elmer Green, Director of the Menninger Foundation voluntary controls projects, was to attach ECG electrodes to the left hand and right ear of an Indian swami, while the swami stopped his own heart. Dr Green thought the swami meant he was going to give himself some kind of neurological shock; but the shock the swami was talking about was psychological.

Before the self-induced shock the swami's recorded heart rate was smooth and even at 70 beats a minute. Suddenly, in the space of one beat, it jumped to almost 300 beats per minute. The polygraph pens jumped up and down five times every second for a span of some 17 seconds.

Animal experiments had shown that it was possible to teach rats to control their hearts, but the swami's experience was the start of a series of experiments to teach humans to learn this technique to cure muscle tension, among other things. Out of this, and similar knowledge derived from the use of curare on rats, was developed the technique of 'biofeedback'.

All learning requires feedback. When learning to speak, it is essential to hear. A child who is hard of hearing speaks poorly, but give him a hearing aid and he may learn to speak like a normal child.

So, by its very nature, biofeedback implies the use of machines. A biofeedback machine is any device that makes a person more aware of a bodily function than he would be normally, and which the person uses in an attempt to control the function voluntarily. A stethoscope can be a biofeedback machine if a person uses it to learn what it feels like to have his heart-rate go up and down and to try to bring his heart under voluntary control.

Biofeedback, as a medical innovation, began in about 1958, the same year as Dr Becker was starting his research into electrical stimulation and regeneration of bone tissue, and about the same time as the Chinese doctors were experimenting with a pulse stimulator for electro-acupuncture use in surgical operations.

But it was a Japanese psychologist, Dr Joseph Kamiya - also in 1958 - who, while studying EEG patterns, began to study in depth what the EEG was recording, what the brain was doing, and what the patient was verbally reporting he felt was happening. He had his subjects sit in a darkened room wired to the EEG and asked them to guess what state they were in: alpha or not alpha, A or B. By the third hour many of the subjects were guessing correctly three times out of four. However, the subjects found it difficult to describe the state. Kamiya said:

'The ineffability of the meditative state so often stressed in mystical writings is similar to statements many of my subjects made; for example: "I can't describe this state ... It has a certain feel about it ...", "I feel calm ..." "I feel stoned ..." "I feel like I'm floating off the chair."'

Unfortunately, biofeedback became the plaything of faddists and cultists and was claimed as the new panacea for everything, but in a few areas the findings have been of real significance. Some of biofeedback's greatest successes have been in relieving muscle tension. With special equipment that registers muscle activity with a tone, or a light, or electronic clicks, it is possible to learn to relax a muscle completely, or to isolate a single motor neuron and learn to 'fire' it at will. Variations on this technique have been used to partially rehabilitate stroke victims, or to eliminate speech defects in slow readers, or to cure facial tics.

A much-publicized technique has been the use of 'alpha-machines', which react to show that the user's brain-waves have entered the 'alpha-state' of calm and relaxation. Brain-waves are a rough measure of mental activity; they are fastest during active, attentive thought, and slowest in deep sleep. Generally, stimulants such as caffeine, tobacco and amphetamines speed up the predominant brain-waves, while alcohol, morphine, marijuana, and decreased blood sugar tend to slow them down.

Put simply, biofeedback is a technique for human self-monitoring in which a person is made conscious of his or her brain-waves while at the same time reflecting on his or her own state of mind; in other words, it is a mechanical device for presenting information externally about what is happening internally so that it may be analysed objectively. The term biofeedback was defined by one of the pioneers, mathematician Robert Weiner, as 'a method of controlling a system by re-inserting into it the result of its last performance'.

With this control the patient can be instructed, among other things, to train himself to enter internal states of consciousness previously only possible to mystics, drug users, or cult initiates. But in less ecstatic circumstances biofeedback is being found an effective therapy in pain clinics for migraine. This is done by means of 'hand or finger-warming exercises'. In practice it is quite easy to learn how to raise the skin temperature of the hands or fingers by simply imagining that they are getting warmer. Soldiers serving in cold climates have been taught this technique. The rationale in migraine is that the headache is caused by dilation of extra- and intra-cranial arteries resulting from excessive autonomic nervous activity. Hand-warming is achieved by relaxation and hence a reduction of sympathetic activity.

But opponents of biofeedback fall back on that good old medical establishment objection to whatever is new, 'the placebo effect', to explain such beneficial responses.

5 In 1946, Dr Grey Walter decided to try imposing new patterns on the existing brain rhythms through the senses. He began by flashing a light at regular intervals into the subject's eyes, and found that this flicker produced a new, strange pattern on the graphs. At certain frequencies the flicker also produced violent reactions in the subject, who was suddenly seized by what seemed to be an epileptic fit.

Grey Walter also noted the similarity of a natural epileptic seizure and one induced by electric shock therapy. He then turned his investigations to normal, resting brain waves of known epileptics, and found that their brain rhythms were grouped in certain frequencies. In order to keep the flicker and the brain synchronized, a feedback system in automatic control was adopted in the form of a trigger-circuit, the flash being fired by the brain rhythms themselves at any chosen time-relation with the rhythmic component of the spontaneous or evoked activity. With this instrument the effects of the flicker were found to be even more drastic than when the stimulus was fixed by an operator, in that in more than 50 per cent of young normal adult subjects the first exposure to feedback flicker evoked transient paroxysmal discharges of the type seen so often in epileptics. He said: 'It was as if certain major chords constantly appeared against the trills and arpeggios of the normal activity.'

He went on to report that the harmonic grouping suggested to him that all that was necessary to get the rhythms to synchronize in a tremendous explosion was an outside coordinator, a conductor who could bring the separate chords together in a simultaneous grand convulsion. A flicker in the alpha-rhythm range, between 8 and 12 cycles per second, acted in just this way on epileptics, provoking them into a seizure at any time. This technique had become a valuable clinical aid in the diagnosis of epilepsy.

In the 1920s a German psychiatrist, Hans Berger, had recorded the first human electro-encephalogram from platinum wires he had pushed into his son's scalp. Berger had surmised that the brain produced only one wave, but he soon discovered that electrodes placed on different parts of the scalp recorded different patterns, indicating various brain waves.

From these investigations there emerged the theory of four basic rhythmic patterns, which were named alpha, beta, delta and theta. The slowest were delta rhythms at a frequency of 1 to 3 hertz, most prominent in deep sleep, theta rhythms had a frequency of 4 to 7 hertz, and were connected with mood; alpha rhythms ran from 8 to 12 hertz, occurring most often in deep meditation; and beta rhythms, between 13 and 22 hertz, seemed to be confined to the frontal area of the brain where complex mental processes take place.

Young children have a tendency to react emotionally to frustration by acts of aggression linked with theta brain waves. It had also been discovered that those adults who were subject to uncontrolled fits of violent aggression often had dominant theta rhythms in their brain waves.

Dr Grey Walter conjectured that this adjustment to frustration and disappointment was 'one of the first and firmest foundations of personality', and went on to say:

> St. Augustine would have been interested in the measure in which EEG records confirm the connection between the sinful mood of the infant and the adult. Few of us indeed escape unscathed from the test. We are all miserable sinners. In ordinary circumstances the theta rhythms are scarcely visible in good-tempered adults, but they seem to be evoked even in them by a really disagreeable stimulus.[334]

6 These observations led to another hypothesis: that the cerebellum is a modulator which arises to the needs of the organism. Cooper speculated, therefore, that chronic cerebellar stimulation leads to a build-up of chemical changes in neurotransmitter systems. If so, a possible eventual reconditioning or normalization of some abnormal brain functions mediated by chemical systems might take place during chronic stimulation of the cerebellar cortex.

7 Another of our colleagues in the Tung Wah Hospital, Dr K. Chau, my physician counterpart, had been experimenting by using the same methods in the treatment of status asthmaticus. He had found that it produced better results than any achieved by conventional therapy. The investigations were conducted from December 1972 to March 1973.

During this period, all 30 cases of bronchial asthma under the care of the medical unit of the Tung Wah Hospital were offered acupuncture and electro-stimulation therapy. Of the patients under observation, six had particularly severe bronchial asthma. They all had had recurrent attacks of severe status asthmaticus, a history of repeated hospital admissions for asthma within the past 12 months, and symptoms that interfered with work and sleep. In all six patients the asthmatic attacks were worse in winter. Four had associated emphysema. Three of them had been under the care of the unit for more than three consecutive years prior to the investigations and had previously received short-term corticosteroid therapy during approximately half of their hospital admissions because of poor response to other treatments. The other three patients had been treated previously in other hospitals, and had come into the unit as emergency cases with severe asthmatic attacks. One of them had continuous asthma for two months before being admitted. Dr Chau also reported his findings in *The Asian Journal of Medicine*:

> All patients showed significant objective response to acupuncture and electro-stimulation therapy for mild to moderately severe

> asthma attacks, and also a significant improvement in the FEVI, FVC and PEFR after treatment ... The results of the present study indicate that in the patients studied, acupuncture and electro-stimulation therapy is superior to conventional therapy in the management of severe bronchial asthma and status asthmaticus. It is superior in the aspects of potency of action, duration of effect, minimum of side effects, and absence of resistance to therapy.[338]

8 Since previous investigations had suggested that monoamines in the brain are especially important in analgesia, the Chinese scientists depleted the test rabbits of monoamines by administering the drug reserpine to block the effect of morphine as an analgesic. Surprisingly, it enhanced the effects of acupuncture. When the monoamines dopamine and 5-hydroxytryptamine were restored to the brain artificially, the effects of acupuncture analgesia returned to normal and morphine was again effective.

Conversely, when they similarly tested the effects of the neurotransmitter substance acetylcholine, they found that it played an important part in acupuncture analgesia. When acetylcholine action was blocked by atropine the effect of acupuncture was very much weakened. Morphine analgesia was not affected by interference with acetylcholine by intraventricular injection of atropine.

9 An American scientist, G. Dauth, reported that in his experimental cerebellar stimulation by implanted electrodes in cats he had concluded, in studying the effects of different frequencies, train durations and pulse durations, that there existed optimal values for each of these parameters, although an increase in pulse duration might compensate for a deficiency in train duration. He also reported that exceeding particular values may provide no greater benefit to the patient. He further suggested that progressively larger currents recruit progressively larger populations of neurons, yet warned against using excessive current application.[70]

Then two researchers, R. R. Myers and R. G. Bickford, demonstrated, in both chloralose and sound-induced myoclonus in cats, that cerebellar stimulation at frequencies of 100–200 hertz clearly suppressed the myoclonus, whereas it was unaffected by stimulation at 1–10 hertz.[69]

10 At first the plates were placed on the anterior lobe alone, because most of the experimental work concerned this area, which is the strongest inhibitor of seizure and motor activity. In certain patients, however, such as those with spasticity, the electrodes were placed only on the posterior lobe, which has strong connections with the motor cortex. Later, all new patients received stimulation of both lobes for better control. Bipolar stimulation between four or more pairs of electrodes was produced simultaneously.

All electrodes on each side were stimulated simultaneously. The current procedure was to stimulate the cerebellum continuously, but in two separate areas alternately. The units had an automatic timer. Stimulation was carried out with rectangular pulses, of 1 msec, with a rate of 7 to 200 hertz, and an intensity of 0.5 to 14 volts. Generally speaking, epileptic patients received stimulation at 10 hertz and 10 volts, and spastic patients 200 hertz and 10 volts, depending on the condition of the patient.

11 One such experiment used 6-hydroxydopamine, which depresses catecholamine biosynthesis and destroys nerve terminals producing a catecholamine. When 6-hydroxydopamine was injected into the cisterna magna of the brains of six rats prepared for electrical stimulation, the rate at which the animals pressed the lever to obtain an electric 'shock' in the medial forebrain bundle was roughly halved. A second injection virtually eliminated self-stimulation in five of the six rats.

Yet another experiment which indicated that noradrenaline is the catecholamine that excited the cerebral reward system of the rat was done with disulfiram and diethyldithiocarbamate. These drugs blocked the conversion of dopamine to noradrenaline. The inhibited self-stimulation of the animals was restored by injecting noradrenaline into a cerebral ventricle.

12 Dr L. S. Illis reported in *Nature*:

> Adult cats were anesthetized with intraperitoneal Nembutal. A catheter in the left ventricle was connected by a two-way tap to normal saline and fixation material. The left fifth lumbar root was exposed by enlarging the root foramen without disturbing the spinal cord dura mater; cardiac pacemaker electrodes were placed around the root and the root was stimulated with a 1 msec pulse, 300 cps, 2.5 volts ... After stimulation of a single posterior root for 65 minutes, *changes were seen in the areas where monosynaptic fibres are known to terminate.*[150] (my italics)

13 In a personal communication with Dr Becker regarding my own research, he said:

> I am enclosing a copy of the paper presented in France and also a preprint of our specific data on acupuncture. Neither of these is up to date and we are vigorously pursuing this line of investigation at the present time. Our additional data, not reflected in either manuscript, has been supportive of our original conception, and I believe at this time I can unequivocally state that there are significant electrical correlations for approximately 50 per cent of the acupuncture points. We have concluded, therefore, that acupuncture has a basis in reality.
>
> Our concept as briefly outlined at the French Symposium is that there is a previously undescribed system of data transmission additional to the nerves in the living organism. We believe that this system is primitive in nature, operates with analog-type DC electrical signals and is concerned with the sensing of injury and effecting its control by healing processes. We believe the system is located in the perineural cells, Schwann cells peripherally and glia cells centrally. There is evidence at least in the glia that these cells are capable of controlling the operational levels of the nerve cells themselves.
>
> In this sense, then, the system becomes analogous to a hybrid computer: that is, with a basic analog system and a superimposed high-speed digital system. Since the input to the system is the sensing of injury, we postulate that this primary system, at least in part, carries the primary pain sensation. Since our data indicate that the system is electronic in nature, and carries messages by means of extremely small currents, the insertion of needles could well produce significant perturbation. Of course, one can theoretically optimize the effect by the direct injection of electrical current.

14 Even microinjections of local anaesthetic into this same area were ineffective in raising the pain threshold; in fact they made the tested animal more sensitive to pain.[147, 265] Researchers observed that the analgesic effect in animals outlasted brain stimulation from a few minutes to several hours, depending on the duration and intensity of the stimulation;[266] in humans the effect lasted up to 24 hours after stopping the stimulation.[2]

It was deduced that stimulation-produced analgesia, like acupuncture, appeared to be modulated by monoaminergic transmission, facilitated by serotonin and dopamine, and antagonized by noradrenaline.[10, 206] Morphine had comparable pharmacological susceptibilities and one noted research scientist suggested that they must both depend, at least in part, upon a common neural substrate. It was also significant that opiate receptor binding sites were found in areas in the brain-stem where SPA was most effective.[178]

15 In pain relief, stimulation of the intralaminar nuclei was analgesic if it remained at low frequency and low amplitude, but increasing the frequency or the amplitude caused arousal, anxiety, and a need to escape, and the pain relief was then totally masked by these emotions. On the other hand, low-level stimulation produced a feeling of relaxation and well-being.[266]

In another demonstration of the importance of frequency, cats were trained to discriminate between two different repetition rates of light-flicker or click. Subsequently, electrodes were implanted in the brain reticular formation, and with bursts of electrical pulses at the same two repetition rates, significant levels of discriminated performance were obtained in all cats very quickly. The memory of what had been learned was to be found in the unique cell-firing rhythm of the brain.[156, 257]

Appendix III
Withdrawal symptoms

Withdrawal

When withdrawn from a user, every psychoactive drug appears, after daily use even for periods as short as one week, to cause a withdrawal or abstinence syndrome (AS).[167, 185]

Apart from opioid withdrawal, the AS may be mild enough to be imperceptible to the physician and cause no complaint by the patient. In addition, there is variation in the severity of the AS in different patients using the same dosages of the same drug. Some who try to withdraw from Valium, for example, experience symptoms more severe than the worst opioid withdrawal; their chronic withdrawal syndrome (CWS) may last as long (or longer) after Valium as it does after methadone withdrawal, that is one and a half years, or longer.[258]

The typical AS for some of the main drugs of abuse are recorded as reported in medical literature.

OPIOIDS

Including codeine, Diconal (dipipanone), Doloxene (dextropropoxyphene - Darvon in US), Palfium (dextromoramide), Fortral (pentazocine - Talwin in US), pethidine (meperidine - Demerol in US), Physeptone (methadone), etc. (listed in order of severity of symptoms).

Craving for the drug of abuse, anxiety, 'yen' sleep, yawning, rubbing nose, rhinorrhoea, lacrimation, perspiration, bone and muscle aches, crossing and uncrossing of legs, muscle twitches, hot or cold flushes, anorexia, gooseflesh, dilated pupils, restlessness, nausea, shivering, stomach cramps, febrile facies, vomiting, diarrhoea, insomnia; increase in respiratory rate, blood pressure (BP), temperature, blood sugar, basal metabolic rate; loss of weight.[174]

The chronic (or protracted) withdrawal syndrome is characterized by a modest decrease in BP, pulse rate, body temperature;

feelings of weakness, apathy, tiredness, social withdrawal, dysphoria. These symptoms persist for at least six months following withdrawal.[201] After methadone withdrawal, it has been reported that the CWS may last for as long as one and a half years.[80]

ALCOHOL

Somatic: gross tremors, muscle jerks, hyper-reflexia. Autonomic: BP increase, heart rate increase, hyperventilation, anorexia, nausea and vomiting, diarrhoea, diaphoresis, fever. Sleep: insomnia (delayed onset and disturbed quality), nightmares. Seizures: major, minor. Sensory: pain, pruritis, visual disturbances, paraesthesias. Affective: anxiety, mania, depression. Sensorium and orientation: agitation, disorientation, delusions, hallucinations. Convulsions may occur 12 to 24 hours after cessation of drinking; one-third of those are likely to go on to full-blown DTs.[290]

BARBITURATES

Barbiturates and related hypnotics such as Seconal, Tuinal and Nembutal; Doriden (glutethimide), Mandrax (methaqualone - Quaalude in US), etc. (Doriden and Mandrax are no longer produced in UK.)

Symptoms commence 12 to 16 hours after the last dose, with anxiety and weakness. After 24 hours a fall in BP, with faintness on standing; tremulousness, restlessness, muscular fasciculations, blepharoclonus (clonic blink reflex),[35] anorexia, vomiting, abdominal distress, mydriasis, hyper-reflexia, insomnia, weight loss, an increased startle response to auditory or visual stimuli. Generalized convulsions (which may occur from the sixteenth hour, till as late as the tenth day after long-acting barbiturates); the incidence is 75 per cent in those using over 900 mg of barbiturate per day for over one month.[305] Reversible psychosis, marked by agitation, insomnia, disorientation in time and place, delusions, auditory and visual hallucinations, elevated temperature, rapid pulse rate, exhaustion. Death can occur.[101] Sleep problems can persist for four months.[166]

TRANQUILLIZERS AND ANXIOLYTICS

Such as Valium, Ativan, Librium, Heminevrin (chlormethiazole - widely used for alcohol withdrawal), etc.

Severe insomnia, tension, restlessness, anxiety, depression, extreme dysphoria, panic attacks, hand tremor, profuse sweating, palpitations, faintness, difficulty in concentrating, nausea, dry retching, vomiting, abdominal pain and diarrhoea, weight loss, breast pain and engorgement, increased thirst with polyuria, blurring of vision, difficulty in focusing, persistent headache and/or head throbbing, muscle pains and 'stiffness', muscle twitching, myoclonic jerks, intolerance to light and sound, sensory changes for touch, noise, vision and smell, metallic taste, paraesthesiae, ataxia, unsteadiness and a feeling of motion, agoraphobia, perceptual disturbance, hallucinations, delusions, depersonalization and feelings of unreality, paranoid thoughts and feelings of persecution, epileptic seizures (a 2.5 per cent incidence recorded among 40 patients who had been using 10 mg diazepam or 4 mg lorazepam daily for at least 4 months and whose dosage was gradually reduced), and influenza-like symptoms lasting from a few days to four weeks. Complete recovery may take a year, or more.[21, 74, 246, 324]

'Following Heminevrin detoxification the patient is likely to experience irritability and sleep disturbance for up to 3 months.'[258] With benzodiazepines, symptoms may subside in about five weeks, but then return in greater severity, even after gradual withdrawal from low doses, and take over two years to subside.[179] Symptoms may even occur for the *first* time several weeks after the last dose, and seizures a few weeks after abstinence.[258]

ANTIDEPRESSANTS

Tricyclics, such as Tofranil (imipramine), or MAO inhibitors such as Parnate (tranylcypromine).

Acute anxiety, restlessness, weakness, nausea, vomiting, diarrhoea, dizziness, disorientation, headaches, confusion, hallucinations, psychosis. Symptoms may persist for several months.[124, 148, 180] Persistent convulsions have been reported in infants born to mothers under treatment with clomipramine (Anafranil).[73]

PSYCHEDELICS

Psychedelics (or hallucinogens) such as PCP or 'angel dust' (phencyclidine), LSD, hashish, marijuana.

PCP AS causes extreme craving, anergia, short- or long-term depression, anxiety, physical discomfort, tremor, insomnia.[231, 310] Marijuana: sleep disturbance, irritability, restlessness, decreased appetite, sweating, sudden weight loss.[317]

STIMULANTS

Such as cocaine, amphetamines, Ritalin (methylphenidate), and various appetite suppressors (Ritalin and Preludin are no longer produced in UK).

A marked 'let-down' effect, extreme fatigue, lengthy sleep, increased appetite, severe cramping of abdominal muscles, symptoms resembling an asthmatic attack, changes in brain-wave patterns, collapse from exhaustion,[35] acute depression.[231]

The feelings of apathy, inadequacy and depression may wax and wane over several months.[100] 'Treatment by antidepressant medication is however best avoided.'[24] Over 10 years of amphetamine use may cause a severe intractable depression on withdrawal.[24] NB: After repeated treatment of rhesus monkeys with high doses of I.V. methamphetamine, the levels of norepinephrine and dopamine in the brain remained markedly reduced for up to six months after the methamphetamine was discontinued.[170]

INHALANTS

Such as solvents and glue.

Psychological dependence occurs regularly but physical dependence is thought to be mild. AS gives fine tremors, irritability, anxiety, insomnia, tingling and cramps of hands and feet, aggressiveness, vertigo, nausea, anorexia, DTs.[61]

NICOTINE

Cigarettes, chewing tobacco, nicotine gum.

Irritability, impatience, headaches, cramps, tremors, energy loss, fatigue,[35] sleepiness, hunger, tenseness, malaise, craving, increase in BP and pulse rate,[118] impairment of memory and concentration.[276]

NB: Two symptoms which occur in withdrawal from *every* group of psychoactive drugs are craving for the substance, and anxiety. Special attention was paid to the effects of NET on these symptoms. The results are detailed on page 155.

Appendix IV
Author's *curriculum vitae*

Margaret Angus Patterson, née Ingram. Born 9 November 1922. MBE, MBChB (Aberdeen), FRCS (Edinburgh).

1944	Bachelor of Medicine and Surgery, University of Aberdeen, Scotland.
1944-5	Rotating internship, Aberdeen Royal Infirmary and Sick Children's Hospital.
1945-7	Residency in surgery in St James' Hospital, Balham, London, under the tuition of Mr Norman Tanner, gastric and oesophageal surgeon.
1948	Fellow of the Royal College of Surgeons, Edinburgh, Scotland.
1948-53	Senior lecturer in Surgery, Ludhiana Christian Medical College, and Surgeon to the College Hospital, Ludhiana, Punjab, India.
1957-61	Medical Superintendent of the Dooars and Darjeeling Tea Association Hospital, and Surgeon to the Hospital, NE India.
1961	Awarded Membership of the British Empire for medical services in India.
1962	Decorated with MBE medal by Her Majesty the Queen in Buckingham Palace.
1964-73	Surgeon-in-charge of the surgical unit of the Tung Wah Group Hospital, Hong Kong (850 beds).
1973-	Consultant in NeuroElectric Therapy for addictions.

Appendix V
Author's publications
(*listed chronologically*)

Patterson MA. Electro-acupuncture in alcohol and drug addictions. Clin Med 1974; **81:** 9–13.

Patterson MA. Acupuncture and neuro-electric therapy in the treatment of drug and alcohol addictions. Aust J Alc Drug Dependence 1975; **2:** 90–5.

Patterson MA. Addictions Can Be Cured. Berkhamsted, England: Lion Publishing, 1975.

Patterson MA. Effects of NeuroElectric Therapy (NET) in drug addiction: an interim report. UN Bull Narc 1976; **28:** 55–62.

Patterson MA. The significance of current frequency in NeuroElectric Therapy (NET) for drug and alcohol addictions. In: Wageneder FM, Germann RH, eds. Electrotherapeutic Sleep and Electroanaesthesia. Graz: R M Verlag, 1978: 285–96.

Capel ID, Williams DC, Patterson MA. The amelioration of restraint stress by electrostimulation. IRCS Med Sci 1979; **7:** 634.

Patterson MA. NeuroElectric Therapy, enkephalin and drug addiction. In: International Review of Opium Studies. Philadelphia: Institute for Study of Human Issues 1981 (in press).

Patterson MA. NeuroElectric Therapy: are endorphins involved? Mim's Magazine 1981; Sep: 22–5.

Capel ID, Pinnock MH, Withey NJ, Williams DC, Patterson MA. The effect of electrostimulation on barbiturate-induced sleeping times in rats. Drug Dev Res 1982; **2:** 73–9.

Capel ID, Pinnock MH, Patterson MA. The influence of electrostimulation on hexobarbital induced loss of righting reflex in rats. Acupuncture and Electro-Therapeutic Res, Int J 1982; **7:** 17–26.

Capel ID, Goode IG, Patterson MA. Tryptophan, serotonin and hydroxyindole acetic acid levels in rat brain following slow or fast frequency electrostimulation. IRCS Med Sci 1982; **10:** 427–8.

Patterson Meg. Getting Off The Hook. Addictions Can Be Cured by NET (NeuroElectric Therapy). Wheaton Ill: Harold Shaw Publishers, 1983.

Patterson MA, Firth J, Gardiner R. Treatment of drug, alcohol and nicotine addiction by NeuroElectric Therapy: analysis of results over 7 years. J. Bioelectricity 1984; **3:** 193–221.

Appendix VI
Chronology of main events that led to the discovery and development of NET

1964

Arrival in Hong Kong. Surgery appointment.

1972

President Nixon's visit to China and worldwide publicity for acupuncture.
Dr Wen visits China to study electro-acupuncture. Electro-acupuncture found to 'cure' drug addictions.

1973

Dr Irving Cooper's visit to Hong Kong which increased my interest in electrical stimulation.
Dr Robert Becker's work with electrical stimulation of bone tissue reported in media.
Reports of Dr Snyder and Dr Pert's discovery of opiate receptors in the brain.
Dr Liebeskind's discovery that pain sensation may be diminished by electrical stimulation of certain areas of the brain in animals.
Treatment of 100 drug addicts in Hong Kong by electro-acupuncture.
Realization that there are significant differences between electro-acupuncture and NET. Decision to concentrate on NET.
Decision to return to London, leave surgery, and research NET in depth.
Establishment of private practice in Harley Street, initiation of research on NET, and application to Medical Research Council for grant to perform double-blind trial of NET. Failure to get sufficient funds.

1974

Treatment of Eric Clapton, with subsequent wide publicity.
Financial support received from rock music groups and Yehudi Menuhin to continue NET research.
Development of first 'Shackman-Patterson' NET stimulators.
Growth of conviction that rapid rehabilitation must follow detoxification. George begins systematic research and programme development.
Intensive investigation of electronics, biology, neuro-electrical stimulation, symptoms, and treatment of addictions to all chemicals producing altered states of consciousness, and their significance.

1975

Visits to European conferences; visit to USA; meeting with Dr Cooper and Dr Becker and with the Institute for the Study of Human Issues.
Shooting for first BBC-TV documentary 'Off The Hook' showing daily treatment of heroin addict and resultant detoxification.
Writing of 'Interim report: addictions can be cured', published in Europe.
Drs Kosterlitz and Hughes's announcement of discovery of endorphins one month after publication of my book.
Visit to Dr Kosterlitz in Aberdeen for discussions regarding electrical stimulation, NET, my 'chemical X' and endorphins.
Rethinking of whole area of treatment of addictions in light of discovery of endorphins and their function.

1976

Research continued; patients treated; different models of machines tested.
Research grants sought in UK and USA.

1977

Filming of second BBC-TV documentary 'Still Off The Hook'.
Treatment of Keith Richards in USA.
Discussions with state (New Jersey) and federal (Washington)

officials regarding use of NET in their clinics. Decision to move to USA.

Showing of second BBC-TV film in UK produces finances for NET clinical trials in UK. Decision to postpone move to the USA.

Development of new Model III of 'Pharmakon-Patterson' stimulator.

1978

Preparations to set up Pharmakon Clinic combining NET detoxification and rehabilitation - the first of its kind anywhere.

Joint research project initiated with Marie Curie Memorial Foundation Research Laboratories to investigate NET in laboratory animals.

Appropriate staff personnel sought and training materials prepared for Pharmakon Clinic.

1979

Preparation of new Model IV NET stimulator for use in Pharmakon Clinic.

Move to Pharmakon Clinic quarters in Broadhurst Manor in Sussex to prepare for patients, negotiate official permits, prepare all paperwork, and ready training programmes.

1980

Clinical trial held in Pharmakon Clinic, January-December.

1981

Commencement of follow-up research of patients treated over seven years in UK.

Departure for USA in March to launch NET there and worldwide.

1982

MEGNET Model V stimulator designed. Work done on materials for publication.

Completion of seven year follow-up research and statistical analysis of findings.

1983

MEGNET Model VI stimulator designed for temporary research purposes.

Arrangements made for the clinical trials at accredited USA universities as required by the Food and Drug Administration of the USA for licensing of the stimulator.

Completion of the MS for *Getting Off The Hook* for publication in the USA, by Harold Shaw Publishers, Wheaton, Illinois.

1984

Advanced MEGNET Model VII stimulator designed. Plans made for NET clinic to be opened in London.

British edition of this book prepared.

MS of counselling book, *The Power Principle*, prepared for publication in the UK.

Appendix VII
Glossary

A layman's glossary of medical terms used in the text (words in italic are defined elsewhere in the glossary).

acetyl choline One of the substances which mediate the transmission of nerve impulses from one nerve to another (e.g. in the brain) or from a nerve to the organ it acts on such as muscles.

acid Slang for LSD, a powerful *hallucinogen* widely, but temporarily, used by most drug addicts. Easily manufactured in illicit laboratories.

ACTH (adrenocorticotropic hormone) It is secreted by the pituitary gland in the brain to maintain *homeostasis* in many body functions. In response to environmental stress, there is increased release of ACTH into the circulation, which in turn rapidly stimulates the cortex of the adrenal gland to secrete more cortisol (or hydrocortisone) which prepares the organism for an emergency.

action myoclonus Spontaneous muscle spasms which occur only with attempted movements.

acupuncture Technique of medical treatment originating in China in which a number of very fine metal needles are inserted into the skin at specially designated points.

adrenaline (epinephrine) Secretion of the medullary (central) part of the adrenal gland in response to strong emotions such as fear or anger, causing an immediate acceleration of bodily functions.

aetiology The cause of a disease or disorder as determined by medical diagnosis.

afferent Directed toward; such as nerve impulses travelling from the periphery of the body inward to the spinal cord.

agonist A drug whose interaction with a *receptor* stimulates the usual biologic response.

alpha rhythms An *EEG* activity of 8 to 12 smooth, regular oscillations per second in subjects at rest.

amyotrophic lateral sclerosis A degenerative disease of the motor neurons causing atrophy of nearly all muscles. It begins in middle age and causes death within two to five years. To date, there is no known treatment.

analgesia Loss of pain sensation without loss of consciousness.

anergy Lethargy or sluggishness.

anaesthesia Loss of pain sensation and also consciousness induced by chemicals.

anode (or **positive electrode**) Electrode by which current enters a device.

antagonist A drug which interacts with the *receptor* but prevents the usual biologic response.

Ativan (lorazepam) A minor tranquillizer of the *benzodiazepine* group. Not available on the NHS by the trade name.

autonomic (nervous system) The division of the nervous system that regulates involuntary action, as of the intestines, heart, etc.

aversive Term used to indicate an adverse response to a drug instead of the usual desired or beneficial effects.

benzodiazepines A group of about ten anti-anxiety drugs or 'minor tranquillizers'. In fact they act by slowing down the entire system. Some are more sedating and have been promoted as sleeping drugs. *Ativan* and *Valium* are the most commonly used by addicts. No longer available on the NHS by their trade names. Have to be prescribed as lorazepam and diazepam.

biofeedback A training technique in which an attempt is made to regulate a body function which is normally involuntary, such as heartbeat or blood pressure, by using instruments to monitor the function and to signal changes in it. Enables an individual to gain some element of voluntary control over autonomic body functions.

cannula A fine tube for insertion into a vein or other body or brain cavity.

catecholamines Cells capable of producing the catecholamine neurotransmitters such as norepinephrine, epinephrine (*adrenaline*), *dopamine*, etc. They affect sleep, memory, food intake, movement, etc.

carbon dioxide (CO_2) bottle-opener A fine tube is pushed through the cork of a wine-bottle and CO_2 forced in from a cylinder under pressure, which results in ejection of the cork.

catatonic A zombie-like condition of unresponsiveness, manifested usually as immobility with extreme muscular rigidity.

cathode (or **negative electrode**) Electrode by which current leaves a device.

cerebral anoxia Lack of oxygen to the brain. This rapidly produces permanent damage to brain functions.

CNS (**central nervous system**) Consists of the brain and spinal cord.

'coke' Cocaine (slang).

'cold turkey' Slang for the condition experienced when coming off *narcotics* such as *heroin* without any replacement drug. Term used because of the 'goose flesh' appearance of the skin.

concha The shell-like area of the ear near the external ear canal.

corpus striatum Part of the basal ganglia of the brain, probably involved in movement control and with perceptual information.

cortical regulation Control of certain body functions by the cortex, or outer surface of the brain.

corticosterone and cortisol (or **hydrocortisone**) Corticosteroids secreted by the cortex of the adrenal glands, which are located on top of each kidney. They influence or control key processes of the body.

cross-tolerance *Tolerance* developed by using one drug, to another drug of a similar pharmacological structure.

cryogenic surgery Surgery by freezing, in which a probe is inserted into the brain and the temperature of the tip is lowered to below freezing-point, destroying the cells causing the pathological condition.

CSF (**cerebrospinal fluid**) A clear fluid which surrounds the brain and spinal cord. Samples for testing (e.g. to measure *endorphins*) are taken by *lumbar puncture*.

cutaneous Pertaining to, or affecting the skin.

Darvon (propoxyphene) A USA pain-killing drug widely abused by drug addicts. Its British equivalent is Doloxene which requires a doctor's prescription but is not a controlled drug. No longer available on the NHS as Doloxene, but must be prescribed as dextropropoxyphene.

decerebrate rigidity Rigidity of the body occurring when brain injury is so severe that it no longer controls the body.

Demerol (meperidine hydrochloride) A USA pain-killing drug, more widely abused in USA than in UK. Known in Britain as pethidine.

diazepam The non-proprietary name for *Valium* et al., and the name by which it has to be prescribed on the NHS.

Diconal (dipipanone hydrochloride plus cyclizine hydrochloride) A pain-killing drug widely abused by addicts and sometimes preferred to heroin. It is now controlled under the Misuse of Drugs Act. Known as Wellconal in USA.

dopamine A substance (catecholamine) produced in the body; its highest concentration is in the basal nuclei of the brain where its function is to convey inhibitory influences to the extrapyramidal system. It is a precursor of *noradrenaline*.

'dope' Marijuana (slang).

double-blind A research programme for testing a new drug or treatment technique where physicians, nurses and patients are all unaware whether patients are receiving active treatment or the inactive *placebo*. Results of the testing are evaluated by scientists who are also unaware of which group received the active treatment and which the placebo. When the programme has been completed, the secret code is broken, and the effects on those who received active treatment are compared with the effects on those receiving inactive placebo.

DTs (delirium tremens) An acute delirium seen in withdrawal from alcohol (or barbiturates). It is characterized by confusion, disorientation, nightmarish hallucinations, gross tremors, high fever, rapid pulse, elevated blood pressure. It peaks three to four days after cessation of drinking.

dysphoria Opposite of euphoria. Used to describe a state of feeling miserable and unwell, without being actually ill.

EEG (electroencephalogram) The recording of the brain's spontaneous electrical output, through several *electrodes* attached to the scalp.

electrode A metal or carbon-rubber conductor which transmits electricity through the skin, such as is used in EEGs or ECGs.

electrolytic Pertaining to electrolysis, which uses a strong electric current to destroy cells.

endogenous Produced from within the body.

endogenous opioids The scientific term used for the *endorphins*, *enkephalins* and dynorphins, to indicate substances manufactured in the brain and elsewhere in the nervous system, which control pain and emotion.

endorphinergic and enkephalinergic neurons Nerve cells which make (and contain and release) *endorphins* and *enkephalins*.

endorphins (A term, used in the text for the sake of simplicity and brevity, to include the group of *enkephalins*.) A family of opioid-like polypeptides found in many parts of the brain and body, which bind to the same *receptors* that bind *exogenous opioids*.

enkephalin The name given to the first '*endorphin*' discovered in 1975. The enkephalins are a group of pentapeptides with a much shorter duration of action than the *endorphins*.

enzyme A protein which acts as a catalyst in certain metabolic reactions, e.g. in breaking down enkephalin in the brain, or alcohol in the liver.

ephedrine A drug whose stimulating effects resemble those of adrenaline and amphetamines. Used mainly to relax the muscles in the bronchi during asthma attacks.

exogenous Supplied from outside the body.

facial or **7th cranial nerve** Controls lacrimation and secretion from the nose and salivary glands, among other functions. Has a sensory connection with the ear.

fistula An abnormal passage from an internal organ to the body surface, or between two internal organs.

Fortral (pentazocine hydrochloride) A pain-killing drug abused by addicts. It must be prescribed by a doctor but it is not a controlled drug. It is known as Talwin in USA. It cannot be prescribed as Fortral on the NHS, but only as pentazocine.

'free-basing' The dissolving of cocaine and the adding of chemical catalysts to precipitate out the pure chemical, which is then smoked. A more potent and rapid effect is obtained than by sniffing cocaine powder up the nose.

GABA (gamma-aminobutyric acid) An amino acid which functions as an inhibitory *neurotransmitter* in all regions of the brain and spinal cord. May have a dual effect on food intake and may also be related to anxiety states. It is deficient in several neuromuscular diseases and perhaps in epilepsy. Also, it may be involved in the diminution of pain brought about by electrical stimulation.

glossopharyngeal or **9th cranial nerve** Carries sense of taste, etc., and is motor to pharyngeal muscles and to the parotid gland. Has a sensory connection with the ear.

'grass' Marijuana (slang).

hallucinogen A chemical substance which causes hallucinations, e.g. LSD, PCP ('angel dust').

hashish A purified extract made from the hemp plant and used as *hallucinogen*.

hepatic Of the liver.

heroin (diacetylmorphine) An opioid prepared from morphine by acetylation. Produces a more powerful 'high' (euphoria) than *morphine*. A normal single dose is 10 mg repeated three or four times daily. An addict commonly uses about 1,000 mg (adulterated, rarely pure) every day, and some have claimed to use up to 10,000 mg daily.

homeostatic Pertaining to homeostasis, i.e. a state of physiological equilibrium produced by a balance of functions and of chemical composition within an organism.

hormones Chemical messengers that are carried in the blood a relatively long distance from their site of production to the area they affect, e.g. insulin, oestrogens, etc.

Hz (hertz) Cycles or pulses per second.

hydration To combine with water.

hypoadrenalism Diminished function of the adrenal glands, e.g. as the result of long-term use of *methadone*.

ictal Relating to a seizure, as in epilepsy.

ictal EEG discharge The firing of neurons caused by a seizure which shows in the *EEG*.

infusion pump A small pump which delivers a constant flow of dissolved drug at a regular rate.

I.V. (intravenous) Injected into a vein. Called '*mainlining*' by addicts.

'junk' Heroin or other opioids commonly abused (slang).

lacrimation Secretion of tears.

laudanum An alcoholic tincture of opium, widely used in Britain in the nineteenth century for relief of pain and discomfort.

ligand The term applied to a molecule which is bound specifically to one site on a protein or nucleic acid.

limbic lobe A part of the brain which deals with memory storage and recall; may also control emotional behaviour such as fear, rage, or motivation.

lorazepam The non-proprietary name for Ativan et al., and the name by which it must be prescribed on the NHS.

lumbar puncture The passing of a long fine needle into the fluid surrounding the spinal cord, in the lower back, to obtain samples of *CSF* for testing, or to inject medication.

mainlining Term used by drug addicts for injection of a drug into their veins.

Mandrax (methaqualone plus an antihistamine, diphenhydramine) A strong sleeping pill, now withdrawn from manufacture in UK. Known as Quaalude in USA and Hyminal in Japan. Widely used as a drug of abuse.

metabolite The substance formed when any natural substance in the body is degraded.

methadone (proprietary name Physeptone) A synthetic *narcotic* which has *cross-tolerance* with *morphine* and *heroin*. It relieves the withdrawal symptoms of heroin addiction without giving the same 'high' (though it is much harder to withdraw from than heroin). Methadone as a syrup or a linctus is widely prescribed for heroin addicts as a maintenance drug in order to reduce drug-related crimes. It is also prescribed as an I.V. injection of Physeptone; each ampoule contains 10 mg of methadone.

morphine A compound extracted from the opium poppy and therefore called an opiate (or *opioid*). It relieves pain, and as a side-effect causes euphoria. Can be chemically altered to the more powerful *heroin*.

myoclonus Spontaneous muscle spasm or jerk.

n Signifies the number of subjects involved in an investigation.

naloxone A specific *antagonist* to all *opioid* drugs. Also an antagonist to the natural *endorphins*; this feature is often used clinically to detect endorphin activity.

narcosis See narcotic.

narcotic Any substance producing stupor associated with pain relief, such as the opiates or synthetic pain-killers.

neurohormone A substance which regulates the function of an organ or a gland by the combined effect of neurologic and hormonal activity.

neuromodulators Natural chemicals which alter neuronal function in various ways.

neuron A nerve cell.

neurotransmitters Chemicals made within the body to carry messages between nerve cells. They bridge the *synapse* and each one has a very specific function. Over 40 have been isolated to date.

noradrenaline (norepinephrine) An important *neurotransmitter* secreted by the medullary (central) part of the adrenal gland and also found throughout the brain and spinal cord. May be involved in the brain's 'reward' system.

opioids (Previously used interchangeably with 'opiates' which referred to opium and its derivatives.) Various sedative *narcotics* containing opium or one or more of its derivatives, such as morphine, heroin, or codeine. The term now includes synthetic compounds having pharmacological effects similar to those of opium.

oral Indicates that a drug is given by mouth.

periaqueductal grey An area of the brain containing many *opioid receptors*.

pharmakon A Greek word meaning drugs, especially those that affect the mind; linked with sorcery in ancient times.

Physeptone Proprietary name for methadone.

placebo An inert substance used as a control in 'blind' experiments to assess the value of a drug or treatment.

post-herpetic neuralgia The severe and often prolonged pain which follows an attack of herpes or 'shingles'.

'pot' Marijuana (slang).

psychotropic The term applied to drugs, normally prescribed by doctors, which affect mood.

receptor A specialized area on the surface of a cell to which either natural substances or *exogenous* drugs attach in order to effect their particular function.

recidivism Relapse to former pattern of behaviour such as substance abuse.

REM sleep Rapid-eye-movement sleep, associated with dreaming. An essential part of normal sleep.

reticular formation An extensive network of nuclei and interconnecting fibres in the central part of the brain which receives *afferent* impulses from many *somatic*, visceral, auditory and visual sensory pathways and relays these impulses to the appropriate areas in the brain. A fully alert state requires this network to be intact.

restraint stress Stress caused by enclosing an experimental animal in a specially designed cage.

RIA (radio-immunoassay) A technique for measuring minute amounts of a substance, based on the use of radioactively labelled antibodies to that substance.

Ritalin (methyl phenidate) A stimulating drug (like the amphetamines) widely abused by addicts, and easily obtained in the black-market.

saline Salt solution. 'Normal saline' is sometimes used as the inert injection in *double-blind* trials.

'scoring' Buying drugs on the black-market (slang).

Seconal (quinalbarbitone) A barbiturate commonly abused by drug addicts.

serendipity The faculty of making fortunate, unexpected discoveries.

serotonin (5HT) An inhibitory *neurotransmitter* whose natural precursor is the essential amino acid, tryptophan. Concerned with functions such as pain, sleep, mood-elevation, aggression, appetite, etc. Lack of it may cause depression and suicidal tendencies.

serum The fluid portion of the blood obtained after removal of the fibrin clot and blood cells.

shakes A coarse tremor of the hands, often seen in alcohol withdrawal. Milder than DTs.

'smack' Heroin (slang).

sniffing or **snorting** The inhaling of a drug up the nose from a special small spoon or through a roll of paper.

somatic Pertaining to the body, as distinguished from the mind.

'speed-ball' Term used as slang in USA to denote conjunction of a depressive and a stimulant drug like 'H and C' (heroin and cocaine).

stereotactic surgery A precise method of destroying a tiny portion of a deep-seated brain structure, located by use of three-dimensional coordinates; as, for example, to relieve the muscle tremors and rigidity of Parkinsonism.

synapse (synaptic junction) The gap between nerve-cells. One *neuron* stimulates another to fire an electrical impulse by secreting a specific *neurotransmitter* into the gap between the cells.

TC **(therapeutic community)** A hostel for the long-term residential treatment of addicts who have stopped using drugs. An average stay is one to two years. They provide structured support of various kinds.

thrombosis Obstruction of an artery or vein by a blood clot forming on the vessel wall.

TM (transcendental meditation) The practice of meditation by means of a 'mantra' or arcane prayer-formula, used by a specific religious cult.

tolerance The need to progressively increase the dose of a drug in order to produce the effect originally achieved by a smaller dose.

transepidermal inductive coupling A receiver is surgically implanted beneath the skin to receive electrical signals from an electrode applied outside that skin area and connected to a special battery.

Tranxene (clorazepate potassium) A minor tranquillizer of the *benzodiazepine* group. This is not available in any form on the NHS.

trigeminal or **5th cranial nerve** Sensory nerve for the face and motor to the jaws.

vagus or **10th cranial nerve** Controls many *autonomic* functions in the body such as the heart rate, breathing and stomach and bowel functions. Has a sensory connection with the ear and the skin behind the ear.

Valium (diazepam) A minor tranquillizer of the *benzodiazepine* group. This is not available on the NHS by the trade name.

vitro (in) A laboratory experiment conducted 'in glass', i.e. outside the living body.

vivo (in) A laboratory experiment conducted in living organisms.

withdrawal The mental and physical symptoms which occur when many types of drug, from heroin to nicotine, have been used regularly for some time and are then discontinued (see Appendix III for details).

Index

Lightning Source UK Ltd.
Milton Keynes UK
UKOW052257171111

182228UK00001B/66/A